NEW CONCEPTS IN INFLAMMATORY BOWEL DISEASE

Edited by **Batool Mutar Mahdi**

New Concepts in Inflammatory Bowel Disease
http://dx.doi.org/10.5772/intechopen.68662
Edited by Batool Mutar Mahdi

Contributors

Rok Orel, Evgen Benedik, Julio Plata-Bello, Silvia Acosta-Lopez, Darja Urlep, Cristiana Popp, Radu Bogdan Mateescu, Kateřina Hokerová, Batool Mahdi

Published by InTech

Janeza Trdine 9, 51000 Rijeka, Croatia

Publishing Process Manager Marina Dusevic
Technical Editor SPi Global
Cover InTech Design team

First published March, 2018
Printed in Croatia
Legal deposit, Croatia: National and University Library in Zagreb

Additional hard copies can be obtained from orders@intechopen.com

New Concepts in Inflammatory Bowel Disease, Edited by Batool Mutar Mahdi
p. cm.
Print ISBN 978-953-51-3845-7
Online ISBN 978-953-51-3846-4

For EU product safety concerns:
IN TECH d.o.o., Prolaz Marije Krucifikse Kozulić 3, 51000 Rijeka, Croatia,
info@intechopen.com or visit our website at intechopen.com.

Meet the editor

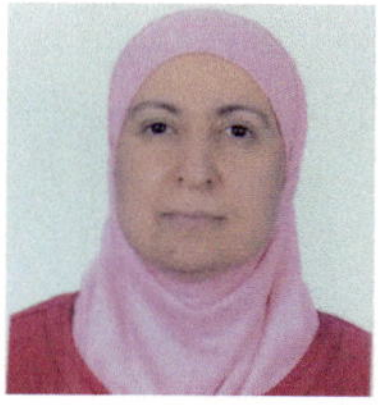

Prof. Dr. Batool Mutar Mahdi is a medical doctor, a Consultant in Clinical Immunology, and the Head of HLA Research Unit, Al-Kindy College of Medicine, University of Baghdad, Iraq. She currently works as a Professor of Clinical Immunology at the same University and holds a master's degree in Clinical Immunology and a board degree in Pathology-Clinical Immunology from Iraqi Board of Clinical Specialization, Iraq, where she has identified the HLA typing of Iraqi population. She has published 70 articles in peer-reviewed journals that were awarded several times and focused on the etiopathogenesis of Inflammatory Bowel Disease; she has written three chapters in books and has given oral and poster presentation at various medical conferences. Prof. Dr. Batool is an international member of the American Society of Histocompatibility and Immunogenetics and other medical societies.

Contents

Preface

This book is a concise review of medically important aspects of inflammatory bowel disease. It covers both clinical and management aspects of this disease in adults. Its two major aims are to assist students preparing for specialty in inflammatory bowel disease and its management and to help people who want to understand more about this condition with brief and flexible sources of information. This book presents the current, medically important information in the rapidly changing field of inflammatory bowel disease. Our goal is to provide readers with an accurate source of clinically relevant information at different levels of medical education. These aims are achieved by utilizing several different formats, which should make the book useful to students and readers with varying study objectives and learning styles. The information is presented succinctly with emphasis on making it clear, interesting, and up to date.

I believe that readers will appreciate a book that presents essential information in readable and interesting formats. I hope this book meets those criteria.

Batool Mutar Mahdi, MB ChB, MSc, FICMS-Path (Clinical Immunology)
Head of HLA (Human Leukocyte Antigens) Research Unit
Department of Microbiology
Al-Kindy College of Medicine
University of Baghdad
Baghdad, Iraq

Section 1

Introduction of Inflammatory Bowel Disease

Chapter 1

Introductory Chapter: Inflammatory Bowel Disease

Batool Mutar Mahdi

Additional information is available at the end of the chapter

http://dx.doi.org/10.5772/intechopen.73512

1. Introduction

Inflammatory bowel disease (IBD) is a collection of inflammatory forms of the colon and small intestine (**Figure 1**).

Under this umbrella is Crohn's disease (CD) and ulcerative colitis (UC) which they are the main types of it. Crohn's disease affects the gastrointestinal tract from the mouth to the anus, whereas ulcerative colitis principally affects the colon and the rectum [1]. A third type of bowel inflammation had emerged known as indeterminate colitis (IC) or inflammatory bowel

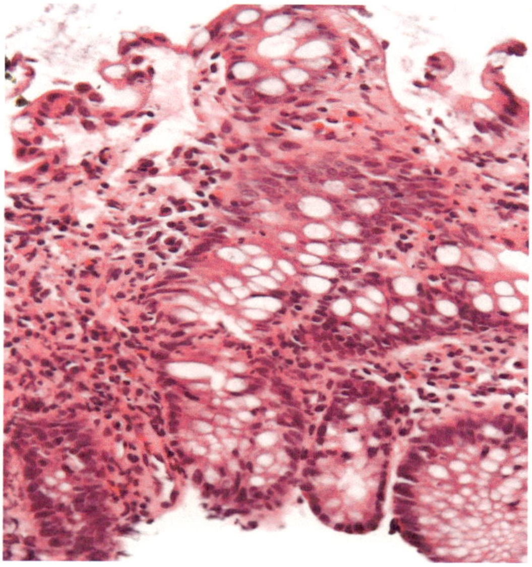

Figure 1. Colonic biopsy of the mucosa shows numerous neutrophils within the crypt and several eosinophils.

disease unclassified (IBDU) when the differentiation between UC and CD is difficult due to the absence of standard golden test that differentiates between these two diseases [2]. IBD can affect any age of the population, but it is more common between 15 and 40 years of age (both young adults and elderly). About 7–20% of IBD patients are children and 60–85% are adults below 40 years of age [3]. There is a bimodal distribution of CD in American cohort population and European and Canadian population; the peak incidence of CD is 15–29 years of age, while the incidence of UC is 20–29 years of age [4]. In smokers, the onset of UC is at later years of age compared to non-smoker patients [5]. Hospital admissions of the patients who were over the age of 65 years of age represent 25% of all hospital admissions for IBD patients [6].

2. Signs and symptoms

Inflammation anywhere along the gastrointestinal tract disrupts the normal mucosal integrity. Thus, IBD can be very painful and disruptive, and it may be life-threatening in some cases. The symptoms are vary from abdominal pain, cramps, swelling in the stomach, recurring or bloody diarrhea, weight loss, tiredness, fever, vomiting, anemia. Other rare symptoms are joint pain, painful red eyes, painful red skin nodules, and jaundice. The characters of these symptoms are remission and relapse [7].

3. Causes

The precise cause is unknown, and it may be due to interaction between environmental and genetic factors leading to immunological responses and inflammation in the intestine.

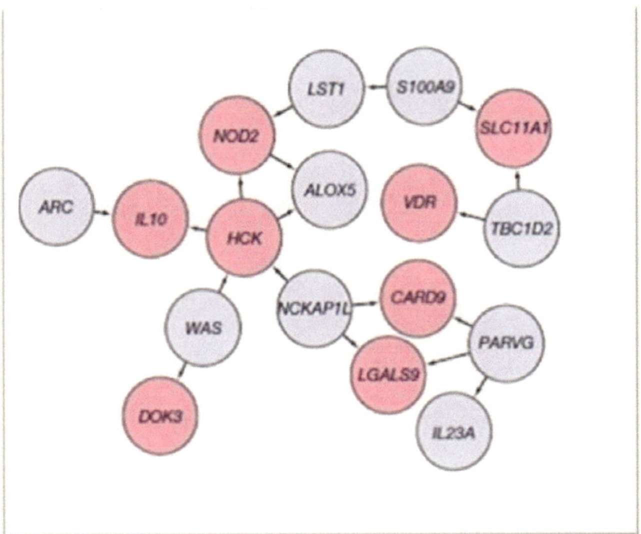

Figure 2. Loci associated with IBD. Pink genes are in IBD-associated loci, blue are not [8].

3.1. Genetic factor

It is more likely to develop IBD if it has a sibling or parent with the IBD. There are about 163 loci that are related to 300 known genes related to cytokine production, lymphocyte activation, and the response to bacterial infection. The most important genes are NOD2, Il10, and CARD9 that had a relation with bacterial interaction and gene HCK which had an important role in anti-inflammation (**Figure 2**) [8].

4. Environmental factors

4.1. Microbiota

The gastrointestinal tract contains many microbiota that maintain normal symbiosis. When there is an alteration in this enteral bacteria may leads to gut inflammation [9]. About 30–50% reduction in *Lachnospiraceae* and *Bacteroides* in the gut of IBD patients and have been prescribed antibiotics for them in the last 2–5 years ago [10]. These drugs in association with other types of food like concentrated milk fat can alter the commensalism bacteria in the gut [11].

4.2. Intestinal barrier

Intestinal epithelial mucosa is an important innate immune mechanism that acts as a barrier preventing microbial gut from invading the epithelial tissue [12]. Changes in intestinal microorganisms lead to uncontrolled immune response that leads to damage this barrier through dysfunctioning of TLR signaling and invading of bacteria initiating an inflammatory immune response [13]. The immune system protects the gut from pathogen like bacteria and virus that leads to inflammation in the digestive tract.

4.3. Diet

The type of diet is an important factor in initiation of IBD [14]. It had been found that animal protein in meat and fish is associated with UC, while plant protein had no effect due to the presence of sulfur-containing amino acid like methionine [15]. Diet containing either intact proteins or free amino acids like elemental, semielemental, and polymeric diets during intestinal inflammation may lead to immunological changes like decrease of serum IgG; increase in the production of IL-6, IL-17A, TGF-β, and IL-10 in the small and large intestines; increase in intestinal permeability; increased number of total and activated CD4+ T helper cells in the small intestine; and proliferating cells in the colon. So, the design of nutritional therapeutic intervention for inflammatory bowel diseases may contribute in the treatment [16]. Eating habit is an important factor in initiation IBD especially in western countries like imbalance in the ratio of n-6/n-3 polyunsaturated fatty acids (PUFAs) in favor of n-6 PUFAs, and a higher ratio of n-6 PUF versus n-3 PUF was associated with an increased UC incidence [17].

5. Risk factors of IBD

5.1. Smoking

Smoking is one of the most important risk factors for developing Crohn's disease but in ulcerative colitis affects non-smokers and ex-smokers. Smoker patients will be affected later on than non-smoker ones [5].

5.2. Ethnicity

Certain ethnic groups like Caucasians and Ashkenazi Jews have a higher risk for developing IBD. Non-Caucasians had more severe disease performance than Caucasians. Non-Central European descent patients who were born in Europe were diagnosed at lower years of age with this disease than those born outside Europe and migrated to The Netherlands [18].

5.3. Age

IBD can occur at any age group, but mainly it starts before the age of 35 [19].

5.4. Family history

Individuals whose parents, sibling, or child have IBD are at a much higher risk of developing IBD. So genetic with epidemiological factors could be used as predictors of the disease course. For example, ileal localization of CD patients was more common in NOD2-variant carriers and IL-6 GC + CC genotypes, identifying C allele as a probable marker of increased risk for ileal CD and earlier onset of the disease in CD patients with a positive family history for IBD. Patients with CD who are TLR4 299Gly carriers are at higher risk for surgery compared with TLR4 299Asp-variant-carrier patients [20].

5.5. Geographical region

Population who live in urban areas and industrialized countries are more liable to develop IBD because they tend to eat more fat and processed food. In addition to that, IBD is more common among people living in northern cold climates. The incidence and prevalence of inflammatory bowel disease show different variations in different geographical regions. IBD is more common in North America and Northern and Western Europe; later on, the incidence was increased in Eastern European and Asian countries [21].

5.6. Gender

IBD affects both sexes equally. Ulcerative colitis is more common among males, while Crohn's disease is more common among females.

6. Complications of IBD

- Malnutrition with resulting weight loss. The frequency of malnutrition in patients with inflammatory bowel disease was high. One of the predictive factors of malnutrition is avoidance of some foods during flares which were associated with higher risk of malnutrition, and many patients had self-imposed food restrictions depending on their beliefs and thoughts [22].

- Colon cancer and other types of tumors. IBD diagnosis at an advanced age had an association with colitis-associated colorectal cancer. Using chemotherapy like thiopurine in older IBD patients leads to an increased risk of non-Hodgkin's lymphoma, nonmelanoma skin cancer, and urinary tract cancers. Furthermore, older age group is accompanied by multimorbidity factors like malnutrition and decreased life expectancy. This needs good cancer screening and medical treatment [23].
- Fistulas or ulcers that go through the bowel wall creating a hole between different parts of the digestive tract that need surgical intervention [24]. The rate of abdominal surgery has decreased and reserved for severe and complicated IBD disease complications due to advances in medical therapy, surveillance, and management methods. The emergency surgery stills in the same rates and increases in surgical recurrence in spite of the reduction in surgical rate morbidity [25].
- Intestinal rupture or spontaneous perforation of the small intestine is rare but can occur in the clinical course of Crohn's disease [26].
- Bowel obstruction. Whether intestinal or colonic obstruction is troublesome for neoplasm as the first clinical manifestation of IBD. This is a clinical thing for surgeons, pathologist, and gastroenterologist to be alert of this. The management of these lesions is surgery like hemicolectomy, segmental colonic resection of the portion involved according to the condition [27].
- Blood loss. One of the complications of IBD is bleeding per rectum or bloody diarrhea that leads to shock [28].

7. Diagnosis

This can be achieved starting from history about chief complain ending with family history. This followed by physical examination and laboratory tests:

1. **Stool sample**: To diagnose the causative microbial agent that causes the disease using fecal samples and assess disease severity. IBD is associated with alteration in the gut microbiota (gut dysbiosis). Bacteria that produce urease leads to transfer of nitrogen to the gut microbiota that is used for amino acid synthesis resulting in a predominance of *Proteobacteria* species and dysbiosis. A possible role for altered urease expression and nitrogen flux in the development of gut dysbiosis suggests that bacterial urease may be a likely therapeutic target for inflammatory bowel diseases [29]. Other fecal tests are S100A12, neopterin, elastase, fecal hemoglobin, alpha-1 antitrypsin, gelatinase-associated lipocalin, chitinase-3-like-1 protein, matrix metalloproteinase-9, lysozyme, M2 pyruvate kinase, myeloperoxidase, fecal eosinophil proteins, beta-defensin-2, and beta-glucuronidase. Some of them had high sensitivity and specificity and correlated with disease activity and response to therapy, and another test is mucosal healing. Fecal calprotectin or fecal lactoferrin is the typical test for assessing IBD activity, even though its specificity and sensitivity are not optimal and it does not have a validated cutoff [30].

2. **Blood test**: There is a panel of blood tests in diagnosis and screening for ulcerative colitis and Crohn's disease like hemoglobin, platelet count, erythrocyte sedimentation rate (ESR), C-reactive protein (CRP), and albumin are widely used [31]. Other laboratory tests have been included like interleukin-1 receptor antagonist, eotaxin, anti-neutrophil cytoplasmic and anti-*Saccharomyces cerevisiae* antibodies, tumor necrosis factor alpha, and thrombopoietin [32–36].

3. **Plain film and barium X-ray (follow-through and enema)**: Plain X-ray can be used when perforation is suspected. Barium X-ray demonstrates the site and the severity of the lesion in the large and small intestine. It also tracks the movement of a thick, chalky liquid barium through the intestines [37].

4. **Flexible sigmoidoscopy and colonoscopy**: This is a direct visualization to sigmoid colon for any ulcers, fistula, and other lesions with biopsy taken. Colonoscopy surveillance is used for early dysplasia detection and treatment, thus preventing progression to colorectal cancer. Techniques and technologies are available to enhance optical diagnosis of dysplasia in inflammatory bowel disease [38].

5. **Capsule endoscopy**: Colon capsule endoscopy is a wireless and simply invasive method for direct visualization of the whole colon and small intestine, screening and monitoring disease activity in inflammatory bowel diseases [39]. The diagnosis of IBD using a pan-enteric video capsule endoscope that visualizes both the small and large bowels is more higher than ileocolonoscopy in patients with active disease [40].

6. **Computer tomography (CT) and magnetic resonance imaging (MRI)**: Used to examine the small intestine and detect any complications of IBD like abscesses, fistulas, and intestinal obstruction. It also excludes other conditions that cause symptoms similar to those associated with IBD like appendicitis. The patient usually drinks an oral contrast, and intravenous contrast may also be injected into a vein prior to the test. Magnetic resonance (MR) enterography has the advantage over other methods of being detection active inflammation noninvasive, lacking ionizing radiation, and demonstrating excellent soft tissue contrast to evaluate patients with inflammatory bowel disease [41].

8. Treatment

1. Anti-inflammatory drugs that decrease inflammation of gut mucosa in spite of its side effect like sulfasalazine and corticosteroids. Sulfasalazine is a sulfa antimicrobial that is used not only to treat IBD that affects gut microbes in the fecal samples by the increasing amount of SCFA-producing bacteria and lactic acid-producing bacteria as well as the decreasing amount of *Proteobacteria* but also to modulate the dysregulated function of the TNBS-induced colitis, increased capacity for carbohydrate metabolism and citrate cycle, and a decrease in the oxidative stress of riboflavin, sulfur, cysteine as well as bacterial pathogenesis like cell motility and secretion, bacterial motility proteins, and flagellar assembly. Furthermore, a higher proportion of *Mycoplasma* concentration [42].

2. Immunosuppressant drugs (immunomodulators): It acts on immune response preventing it from attacking the bowel and causing inflammation like anti-TNF antibodies (infliximab)

(IFX). Some patients will respond to this treatment, while others will not. The transmembrane TNF-α might be linked to response to IFX by promoting reverse signaling-induced apoptosis in inflammatory cells. The percentage of tmTNF-α bearing lymphocytes and monocytes and the intensity of tmTNF-α in the circulating leukocyte were directly related to primary response to IFX. Immunosuppressants have many side effects including rashes and infections [43].

3. **Antibiotics**: The pathogenesis of inflammatory bowel disease is complex and involves the interaction between genetic and environmental factors. One modality is prescription of antibiotic like oral vancomycin with or without gentamicin that targets and kill Gram-negative and anaerobic bacteria that may trigger or aggravate IBD symptoms [44].

4. **Antidiarrheal drugs and laxatives**: Diarrhea is a common clinical symptom of inflammatory bowel diseases with abdominal pain, urgency, and fecal incontinence. The pathophysiology of it is due to a defect in absorption of salt and water by the inflamed bowel with inflammation. So, one mode of treatment is antidiarrheal drugs to treat IBD symptoms [45].

5. **Lifestyle choices**: IBD is increased in both developed and developing countries due to lifestyle which is important in patients with IBD like obesity which is increased in parallel with IBD. The possible cause is due to adipose tissue that produces pro-inflammatory adipokines and provides a possible mechanism for the links between obesity and IBD. Other possible methods of lifestyle are drinking plenty of fluids, which helps to compensate for those lost in stool, and vitamin and mineral supplements, which can help in patients with nutritional deficiencies. Avoiding dairy products and stressful situations also improves symptoms. Exercising and quitting smoking can improve the IBD [46].

6. Surgery can sometimes be necessary for people with IBD, like strictureplasty, to widen a narrowed bowel, closure or removal of fistulas, removal of affected portions of the intestines, and removal of the entire colon and rectum, for severe cases of ulcerative colitis [47].

8.1. Prevention

The hereditary causes of IBD cannot be prevented. However, you may be able to reduce your risk of developing IBD or prevent a relapse [48]. This can be achieved by eating healthy foods like regular consumption of extra virgin olive oil, which is the main source of fat in the Mediterranean diet [49]. Other methods are exercising regularly and quit smoking. In addition to that, using infliximab helps to prevent recurrence [50].

Author details

Batool Mutar Mahdi

Address all correspondence to: abas_susan@yahoo.com

HLA Research Unit, Department of Microbiology and Immunology, Al-Kindy College of Medicine, University of Baghdad, Iraq

References

[1] Baumgart DC, Carding SR. Inflammatory bowel disease: Cause and immunobiology. The Lancet. 2007;**369**:1627-1640

[2] Mahdi BM. A review of inflammatory bowel disease unclassified—indeterminate colitis. Journal of Gastroenterology and Hepatology Research. 2012;**1**:241-246

[3] Prelipcean CC, Mihai C, Gogalniceanu P, Mihai A. What is the impact of age on adult patients with inflammatory bowel disease? Clujul Medical. 2013;**86**:3-9

[4] Johnston RD, Logan RF. What is the peak age for onset of IBD? Inflammatory Bowel Diseases. 2008;**14**(Suppl 2):S4-S5

[5] Lakatos PL, Szamosi T, Lakatos L. Smoking in inflammatory bowel disease: Good, bad or ugly? World Journal of Gastroenterology. 2007;**13**:6134-6139

[6] Bucharan J, Wordsworth S, Tariq A, et al. Managing the long term care of inflammatory bowel disease patients: The cost to European healthcare providers. Journal of Crohn's and Colitis. 2011;**5**:306-316

[7] Wang GF, Ren JA, Liu S, Chen J, Gu GS, Wang XB, Fan CG, Li JS. Clinical characteristics of non-perianal fistulating Crohn's disease in China: A single-center experience of 184 cases. Chinese Medical Journal. 2012;**125**:2405-2410

[8] Jostins L, Ripke S, Weersma RK, Duerr RH, DP MG, Hui KY, et al. Host-microbe interactions have shaped the genetic architecture of inflammatory bowel disease. Nature. 2012; **491**:119-124

[9] Mukhopadhya I, Hansen R, El-Omar EM, Hold GL. IBD—What role do proteobacteria play? Nature Reviews Gastroenterology & Hepatology. 2012;**9**:219-230

[10] Aroniadis OC, Brandt LJ. Fecal microbiota transplantation: Past, present and future. Current Opinion in Gastroenterology. 2013;**29**:79-84

[11] Kotanko P, Carter M, Levin NW. Intestinal bacterial microflora—A potential source of chronic inflammation in patients with chronic kidney disease. Nephrology, Dialysis, Transplantation: Official Publication of the European Dialysis and Transplant Association—European Renal Association. 2006;**21**:2057-2060

[12] Maloy KJ, Fiona P. Intestinal homeostasis and its breakdown in inflammatory bowel disease. Nature. 2011;**474**:298-306

[13] Cario E. Toll-like receptors in inflammatory bowel diseases: A decade later. Inflammatory Bowel Diseases. 2010;**16**:1583-1597

[14] Vibeke A, Anja O, Franck C, Anne T, Ulla V. Diet and risk of inflammatory bowel disease. Digestive and Liver Disease. 2012;**44**:185-194

[15] Magee EA, Richardson CJ, Hughes R, Cummings JH. Contribution of dietary protein to sulfide production in the large intestine: An in vitro and a controlled feeding study in humans. The American Journal of Clinical Nutrition. 2000;**72**:1488-1494

[16] Souza AL, Fiorini Aguiar SL, Gonçalves Miranda MC, Lemos L, Freitas Guimaraes MA, Reis DS, Vieira Barros PA, Veloso ES, Carvalho TG, Ribeiro FM, Ferreira E, Cara DC, Gomes-Santos AC, Faria AMC. Consumption of Diet Containing Free Amino Acids Exacerbates Colitis. 2017

[17] Scaioli E, Liverani E, Belluzzi A. The imbalance between n-6/n-3 polyunsaturated fatty acids and inflammatory bowel disease: A comprehensive review and future therapeutic perspectives. International Journal of Molecular Sciences. 2017;**18**. pii: E2619

[18] Spekhorst LM, Severs M, de Boer NKH, Festen EAM, Fidder HH, Hoentjen F, Imhann F, de Jong DJ, van der Meulen-de Jong AE, Pierik MJ, van der Woude CJ, Dijkstra G, Ponsioen CY, Löwenberg M, Oldenburg B, Weersma RK. The impact of ethnicity and country of birth on inflammatory bowel disease phenotype: A prospective cohort study. Journal of Crohn's & Colitis. 2017;**11**:1463-1470

[19] Stallmach A, Hagel S, Gharbi A, et al. Medical and surgical therapy of inflammatory bowel disease in the elderly—Prospects and complications. Journal of Crohn's and Colitis. 2011;**5**:177-188

[20] Dragasevic S, Stankovic B, Milosavljevic T, Sokic-Milutinovic A, Lukic S, Alempijevic T, Zukic B, Kotur N, Nikcevic G, Pavlovic S, Popovic D. Genetic and environmental factors significant for the presentation and development of inflammatory bowel disease. European Journal of Gastroenterology & Hepatology. 2017;**29**:909-915

[21] Vegh Z, Kurti Z, Lakatos PL. Epidemiology of inflammatory bowel diseases from west to east. Journal of Digestive Diseases. 2017;**18**:92-98

[22] Casanova MJ, Chaparro M, Molina B, Merino O, Batanero R, Dueñas-Sadornil C, et al. Prevalence of malnutrition and nutritional characteristics of patients with inflammatory bowel disease. Journal of Crohn's & Colitis. 2017;**11**:1430-1439

[23] Taleban S, Elquza E, Gower-Rousseau C, Peyrin-Biroulet L. Cancer and inflammatory bowel disease in the elderly. Digestive and Liver Disease. 2016;**48**:1105-1111

[24] Makris GM, Charalampopoulos A, Siristatidis C, Fexi D, Chrelias C, Battista MJ, Papantoniou N. Y-type anovulvar fistula complicating inflammatory bowel disease. The American Surgeon. 2016;**82**:305-307

[25] Toh JWT, Wang N, Young CJ, Rickard MJFX, Keshava A, Stewart P, Kariyawasam V, Leong R. Major abdominal and perianal surgery in Crohn's disease: Long-term follow-up of Australian patients with Crohn's disease. Diseases of the Colon and Rectum. 2018; **61**:67-76

[26] Freeman HJ. Spontaneous free perforation of the small intestine in Crohn's disease. Canadian Journal of Gastroenterology. 2002;**16**:23-27

[27] Romero C, Sirsi S, Asarian A, Levine J, Xiao P. Giant inflammatory polyposis, a phenomenon of inflammatory bowel disease, presenting as acute large bowel obstruction mimicking colonic neoplasm. Journal of Surgery Case Reports. 2017;**7**:rjx174

[28] Jehangiri AU, Gul R, Hadayat R, Khan AN, Zabiullah KL. Causes of lower gastrointestinal bleeding on colonoscopy. Journal of Ayub Medical College, Abbottabad. 2017;**29**:468-471

[29] Ni J, Shen TD, Chen EZ, Bittinger K, Bailey A, Roggiani M, Sirota-Madi A, Friedman ES, Chau L, Lin A, Nissim I, Scott J, Lauder A, Hoffmann C, Rivas G, Albenberg L, Baldassano RN, Braun J, Xavier RJ, Clish CB, Yudkoff M, Li H, Goulian M, Bushman FD, Lewis JD, Wu GD. A role for bacterial urease in gut dysbiosis and Crohn's disease. Science Translational Medicine. 2017;**15**. pii: eaah6888

[30] Di Ruscio M, Vernia F, Ciccone A, Frieri G, Latella G. Surrogate fecal biomarkers in inflammatory bowel disease: Rivals or complementary tools of fecal calprotectin? Inflammatory Bowel Disease. 2017;**19**:78-92

[31] Oh K, Oh EH, Baek S, Song EM, Kim GU, Seo M, Hwang SW, Park SH, Yang DH, Kim KJ, Byeon JS, Myung SJ, Yang SK, Ye BD. Elevated C-reactive protein level during clinical remission can predict poor outcomes in patients with Crohn's disease. PLoS One. 2017;**12**:e0179266

[32] Propst A, Propst T, Herold M, et al. Interleukin-1 receptor antagonist in the differential diagnosis of inflammatory bowel diseases. European Journal of Gastroenterology & Hepatology. 1995;**7**:1031-1036

[33] Chen W, Paulus B, Shu D, et al. Increased serum levels of eotaxin in patients with inflammatory bowel disease. Scandinavian Journal of Gastroenterology. 2001;**36**:515-520

[34] Papadakis KA, Targan SR. Serologic testing of inflammatory bowel disease: Its value in indeterminate colitis. Current Gastroenterology Reports. 1999;**1**:482-485

[35] Komatsu M, Kobayashi D, Saito K, et al. Tumor necrosis factor-alpha in serum of patients with inflammatory bowel disease as measured by a highly sensitive immuno-PCR. Clinical Chemistry. 2001;**47**:1297-1301

[36] Kapsoritakis AN, Potamianos SP, Sfiridaki AI, et al. Elevated thrombopoietin serum levels in patients with inflammatory bowel disease. The American Journal of Gastroenterology. 2000;**95**:3478-3481

[37] O'Connor OJ, McSweeney SE, McWilliams S, O'Neill S, Shanahan F, Quigley EM, Maher MM. Role of radiologic imaging in irritable bowel syndrome: Evidence-based review. Radiology. 2012;**262**:485-494

[38] Beintaris I, Rutter M. Advanced imaging in colonoscopy: Contemporary approach to dysplasia surveillance in inflammatory bowel disease. Frontline Gastroenterology. 2016; **7**:308-315

[39] Muguruma N, Tanaka K, Teramae S, Takayama T. Colon capsule endoscopy: Toward the future. Clinical Journal of Gastroenterology. 2017;**10**:1-6

[40] Leighton JA, Helper DJ, Gralnek IM, Dotan I, Fernandez-Urien I, Lahat A, Malik P, Mullin GE, Rosa B. Comparing diagnostic yield of a novel pan-enteric video capsule endoscope with ileocolonoscopy in patients with active Crohn's disease: A feasibility study. Gastrointestinal Endoscopy. 2017;**85**:196-205

[41] Yoon HM, Suh CH, Kim JR, Lee JS, Jung AY, Kim KM, Cho YA. Diagnostic performance of magnetic resonance enterography for detection of active inflammation in children and adolescents with inflammatory bowel disease: A systematic review and diagnostic meta-analysis. JAMA Pediatrics. 2017;**171**:1208-1216

[42] Zheng H, Chen M, Li Y, Wang Y, Wei L, Liao Z, Wang M, Ma F, Liao Q, Xie Z. Modulation of gut microbiome composition and function in experimental colitis treated with sulfasalazine. Frontiers in Microbiology. 2017;**8**:1703

[43] Amini Kadijani A, Asadzadeh Aghdaei H, Sorrentino D, Mirzaei A, Shahrokh S, Balaii H, Nguyen VQ, Mays JL, Reza Zali M. Transmembrane TNF-α density, but not soluble TNF-α level, is associated with primary response to infliximab in inflammatory bowel disease. Clinical and Translational Gastroenterology. 2017;**8**:e117

[44] Lev-Tzion R, Ledder O, Shteyer E, MLN T, Uhlig HH, Turner D. Oral vancomycin and gentamicin for treatment of very early onset inflammatory bowel disease. Digestion. 2017; **95**:310-313

[45] Wenzl HH. Diarrhea in chronic inflammatory bowel diseases. Gastroenterology Clinics of North America. 2012;**41**:651-675

[46] Harper JW, Zisman TL. Interaction of obesity and inflammatory bowel disease. World Journal of Gastroenterology. 2016;**22**:7868-7881

[47] Delaney JD, Holbrook JT, Dewar RK, Laws PJ, Engel AF. Frequency of equivocation in surgical meta-evidence: A review of systematic reviews within IBD literature. BMJ Open. 2017;**7**:e018715

[48] Cohen-Mekelburg S, Schneider Y, Gold S, Scherl E, Steinlauf A. Risk stratification for prevention of recurrence of postoperative Crohn's disease. Gastroenterology & Hepatology. 2017;**13**:651-658

[49] Santangelo C, Vari R, Scazzocchio B, De Sanctis P, Giovannini C, D'Archivio M, Masella R. Anti-inflammatory activity of extra virgin olive oil polyphenols: Which role in the prevention and treatment of immune-mediated inflammatory diseases? Endocrine, Metabolic & Immune Disorders Drug Targets. 2017;**13**

[50] Regueiro M, Schraut W, Baidoo L, et al. Infliximab prevents Crohn's disease recurrence after ileal resection. Gastroenterology. 2009;**136**:441-450

Section 2

Histopathology of Inflammatory Bowel Disease

Histologic Features with Predictive Value for Outcome of Patients with Ulcerative Colitis

Cristiana Popp and Radu Bogdan Mateescu

Additional information is available at the end of the chapter

http://dx.doi.org/10.5772/intechopen.72893

Abstract

Ulcerative colitis is an inflammatory bowel disease with variable evolution, in which is difficult to establish patient's outcome. Histology is an important part of diagnosis of ulcerative colitis and has an increasing role in patients' management, since increasingly more histologic features with predictive value are being identified and validated. This chapter presents the most important histologic prognostic factors that should be included in histologic reports of patients with ulcerative colitis. Basal plasmacytosis and histologic healing are the most significant validated factors of prognosis in ulcerative colitis, while dysplasia is important since colorectal carcinoma is a severe complication of the disease.

Keywords: ulcerative colitis, predictive value, prognosis, histologic factors, basal plasmacytosis, dysplasia, histologic scores, histologic healing

1. Introduction

Inflammatory bowel diseases (IBD) are a group of chronic diseases with an unpredictable evolution, with repeated flare-ups and remissions. The most important inflammatory bowel diseases are ulcerative colitis and Crohn's disease.

One of the most difficult problems of management of patients with inflammatory bowel disease is the prognosis of these patients. This is an important issue for patients, since their life is involved; for medical specialists, who should choose the best therapeutical approach and surveillance schedule; for the health insurance system, which should tailor costs according to patient's needs and for the society, since patients with IBD are young and are facing a lifetime of partial disability and medical dependence.

This chapter aims to describe histologic features with prognostic significance in ulcerative colitis (UC). Usually, patients with UC undergo multiple colonoscopies with biopsies for diagnosis and surveillance. The European consensus on the histopathology of inflammatory bowel disease recommends for diagnosis to harvest at least two biopsies from minimum five sites along the colon, including the rectum and the terminal ileum, and for surveillance four biopsies from every 10 cm of the colon [1]. Routinely reporting histologic features with prognosis values is an important component of management of these patients.

2. Histologic diagnosis of ulcerative colitis

Histologic diagnosis of UC requires examination of multiple colonic biopsies, including ones from the rectum and the terminal ileum, accompanied by clinical and endoscopical data [1].

Classical histologic features of untreated UC can be divided into three categories:

a. Inflammatory lesions: characteristic pattern is chronic active colitis with polymorphous inflammatory infiltrate in lamina propria and variable intraepithelial extension of neutrophils with or without ulcerations [2]. Activity is defined by the presence of neutrophils in lamina propria, in crypt epithelium (cryptitis) and inside crypt lumina (crypt abscesses) [3]. Chronicity is defined by lymphoplasmacytosis of lamina propria, with variable basal plasmacytosis instead of plasma cell gradient [2–4].

b. Architectural changes: including distortion of crypts' architecture, cryptic atrophy and villous aspect of superficial epithelium [1]. In normal large bowel mucosa, crypts are evenly distributed, parallel, with similar length (in accordance with the site of the biopsy). Architectural distortion in UC includes shortening and branching of crypts, separated by unequal spaces. Also, there is a variable hyperplasia of muscularis mucosa (especially in long-standing disease). Although architectural distortion is variable in time, it is found in all patients with UC, even during remission periods [5].

c. Cellular changes: including Paneth cell metaplasia, mucin depletion, regenerative epithelial changes and dysplastic epithelial changes. Paneth cells are normal in proximal colon, but finding them in the distal colon and in the rectum is a sign of repeated processes of ulceration repair and epithelial regeneration [6]. Although nonspecific, Paneth cell metaplasia is suggestive of a long-standing ulcerative colitis [7]. Paneth cells are involved in innate and acquired local immunity and can be modulators of inflammation and repair in UC [8]. Mucin depletion is the reduction of number of goblet cells and/or the decrease of the quantity of mucin in their cytoplasm [7]. It is not a diagnosis change, being correlated with inflammation and regeneration [7]. Dysplasia in UC is a late event and has a great significance for patients' outcome. It will be discussed later.

3. Histologic features with prognosis value in UC

Although prognosis is always an important challenge in management of chronic diseases, reporting prognosis factors in UC is, somehow, a new target for pathologists. There are three issues that should be accomplished for a histologic feature to become a used prognosis factor: validated predicting value, high intra- and interobserver agreement and wide applicability.

Multiple histologic and immunohistochemical features were proposed to be used in current practice, but only some are properly studied and validated. None of these features is reliable by itself; so, probably histologic prognosis factors will be better used in a composite score, including clinical, endoscopical and serologic features [9, 10].

Some of the most important histologic features involved in establishing prognosis in UC are as follows:

3.1. Basal plasmacytosis

Basal plasmacytosis (**Figure 1**) represents the presence of plasma cells in the lower part of the mucosa, between the base of the crypts and muscularis mucosae [11]. Rectal basal plasmacytosis is the most used microscopic lesion as prognosis factor, confirmed and validated by several studies [10–12]. Basal plasmacytosis is an early feature, frequently found in patients with UC, being used in diagnosis [12]. Its presence on rectal biopsies taken during remission has a strong value in predicting short-time relapse of the disease, especially if there is an increase of severity of basal plasmacytosis in asymptomatic patients [11, 13]. Although a recent study failed to demonstrate the value of basal plasmacytosis as prognosis factor [14], it is included in most recent ECCO-ESP European consensus on histopathology of inflammatory bowel disease as predictive of ensuing clinical relapse [1]. It fulfills all three conditions for a good predictive factor, because it was validated in some independent case series and cohort studies, has a very good reproducibility and a wide applicability, since it can be evaluated on routine histologic slides.

3.2. High number of eosinophils

The presence of eosinophils (**Figure 2**) is usually associated with basal plasmacytosis. Eosinophils are not simple effectors in UC but active players in inflammation and mucosal repair [12, 15].

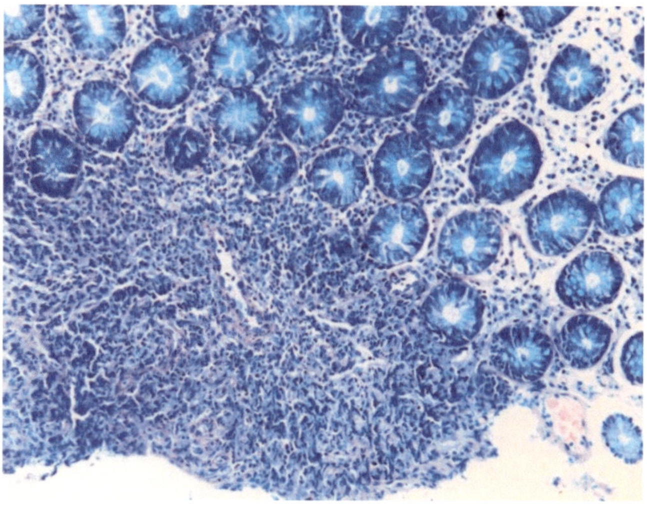

Figure 1. Basal plasmacytosis in a newly diagnosed patient with UC (Giemsa, 200×).

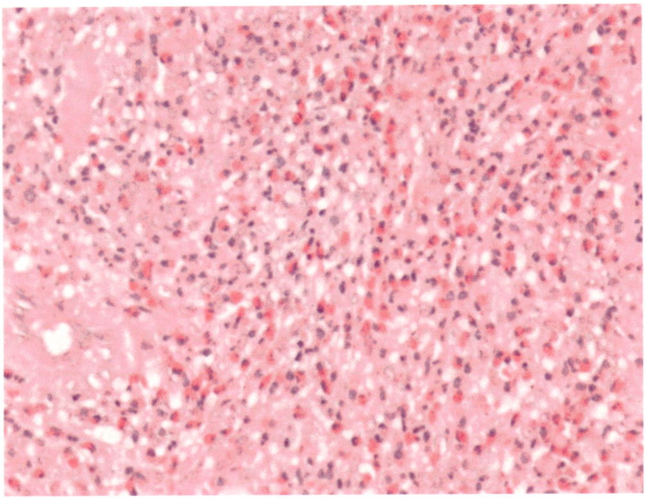

Figure 2. Numerous eosinophils in lamina propria in a patient with active UC. The area is in the immediate vicinity of an ulceration (hematoxylin & eosin, 100×).

Persistence of eosinophils in lamina propria after clinical remission indicates a high risk of relapse [1, 11], and some studies demonstrated that in quiescent phase of UC, remaining eosinophils are activated [16]. Their exact role is not fully understood, but they seem to be involved in plasma cell survival [12], to have proinflammatory and promotility effects [15] and to participate in normal and pathological repair of the mucosa [16]. Some studies demonstrated that high number of eosinophils is associated with a poor response to therapy [17], an increased incidence of relapse [18] and a high risk of extensive fibrosis and stenosis [12]. Reporting the number of eosinophils in UC patients can be done semi-quantitatively and this can be a good predictive factor if more studies will validate it.

3.3. Cryptitis and crypt abscesses

Cryptitis is the extension of neutrophils in the epithelium of crypts, while crypt abscesses are accumulations of neutrophils in the lumina of the crypts (**Figure 3**). They are, both, identified in active phase of UC [2]. They are predictive for an aggressive, refractory disease especially in older patients [19]. One study identified cryptitis in the majority of relapsing patients, while none of the non-relapsers had this feature on the initial biopsy [18]. The presence of cryptitis and crypt abscesses is a histologic feature with high reproducibility and wide applicability, but needs further studies to validate it as a valuable predictive factor.

3.4. Histologic activity

It is usually evaluated using a semi-quantitative score. The most frequently used in UC is Geboes score, which is a histologic scale including data about active inflammation and chronicity changes [20]. Although there are studies that validated Geboes score as a predictive marker in UC [10, 21], it is difficult to use in current practice because there are too many parameters to be quantified, some of them having a poor reproducibility. Also, interobserver

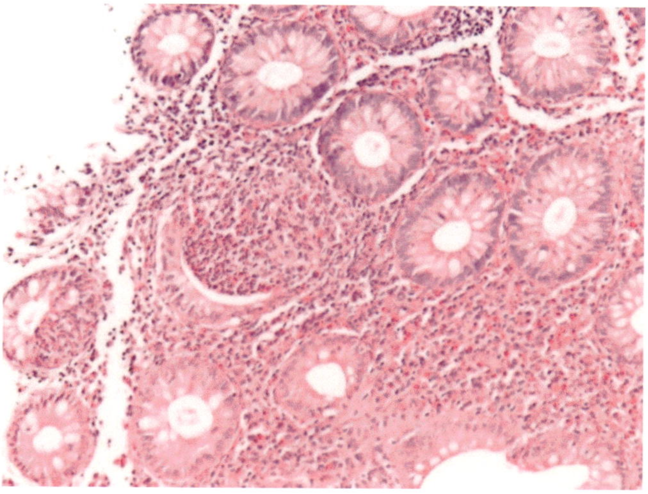

Figure 3. Cryptitis and cryptic abcess in a patient with active UC in the first relapse after initiating therapy (hematoxylin & eosin, 100×).

agreement varies among studies, being probably responsible for contradictory results. A Simplified Geboes Score is also available, being developed and validated with similar results as the original score [22].

Recently, some other promising scores for UC have been validated and used in current practice, the most prominent being Nancy and Robarts Indexes [23, 24]. They have a good reproducibility and a wider accessibility, but they still need validation as predictive tools for UC [25]. Nancy Index assesses, in a sequential form, the presence of ulceration, acute inflammatory infiltrate (presence of neutrophils and eosinophils in lamina propria and in epithelium) and chronic inflammatory infiltrate, using a semi-qualitative scale very easy to understand, which allows a great reproducibility [23]. All features have demonstrated their predictive value for relapse in different studies, so we have a good probability for Nancy Index to have an acceptable predictive value. It is recommended that Nancy Index be used in current practice; a fact that will ease further studies for validating this index [26]. Robarts Index is considered to be validated for UC diagnosis, but data are still lacking about its predictive value for UC outcome. Robarts score includes evaluation of: chronic inflammatory infiltrate, activity and the severity of erosions or ulceration [26]. Since it is more difficult to use, probably it is more suitable for clinical trials and research studies [27].

3.5. Architectural distortion

Distortion of crypt architecture (**Figure 4**) is usually present on colonic biopsies in patients with UC, even in cases with complete remission. It is the result of repeated episodes of inflammation, ulceration and repair and is the witness of mucosal remodeling. Architectural distortion includes shortening and branching of the crypts with inequality of inter-crypt distance [2]. Severe architectural distortion in a predictive factor for a short-time relapse in patients with clinical remission of UC [28]. Also, worsening of architectural distortion in

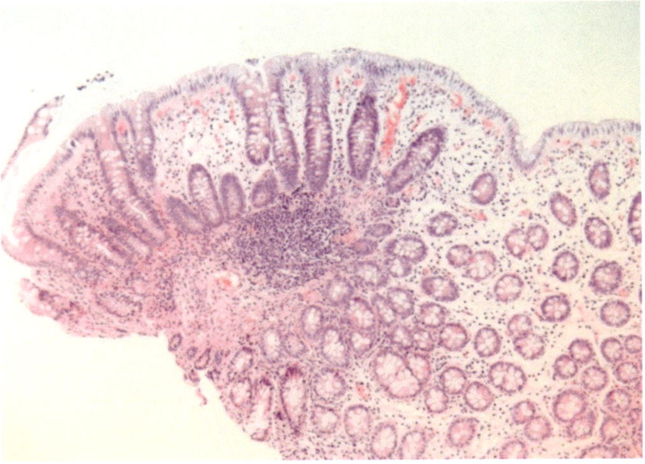

Figure 4. Architectural distortion of colonic mucosa in a patient with long-standing UC. Note an unequal distance between crypts and lack of crypt parallelism. Also, although there is no activity, some inflammation persists (hematoxylin & eosin, 40×).

patients with UC without an intervening acute inflammatory episode is usually a good predictor of evolution toward dysplasia, correlating with acquisition of mutations in epithelial cells [29].

3.6. Paneth cell metaplasia

Presence of Paneth cells (**Figure 5**) in the base of the crypts beyond splenic flexure is considered pathologic in UC. Their role and importance are still understudied. Paneth cell metaplasia

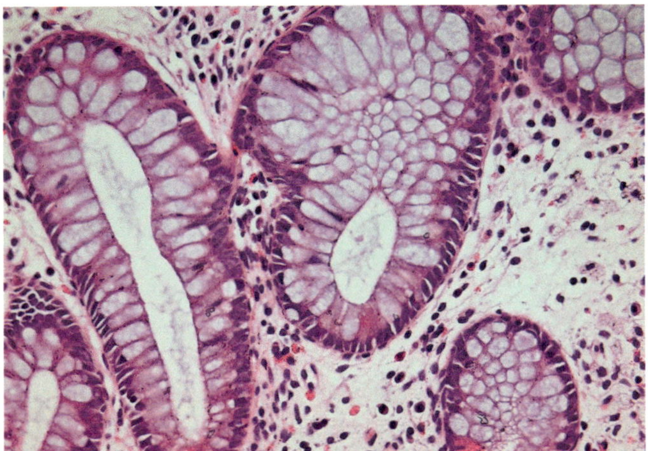

Figure 5. Paneth cells in the base of the crypts on a rectal biopsy, in a patient with a long-standing ulcerative colitis and minimal inflammation of rectal mucosa (hematoxylin & eosin 200×).

is considered a response to chronic injury and is identified in patients with long evolution of the disease, indicating their evolution toward malignant epithelial lesions [30, 31]. Practically, after ulceration, mucosa is repaired by various clones of epithelial cells; some of them with anomalies that make them differentiate as Paneth cells. In areas of Paneth cell metaplasia without dysplasia, there were identified mutations of β-catenin similar to those in dysplastic and malignant lesions of colon [31].

Paneth cells are involved in innate immunity of the gut, secreting antimicrobial proteins [8]. In inflammatory bowel disease, they probably are involved in offering antibacterial protection for the damaged mucosa [8]. It is still unknown if the defensins produced by Paneth cells are involved in the abnormal response of local immunity in UC [32].

3.7. Dysplasia

Dysplasia represents the morphologic changes of epithelial cells that are indicating accumulation of DNA damage and progression toward malignancy. Carcinogenesis in UC is inflammation-driven and has a different pathway than usual colorectal carcinogenesis. Epithelial cells are acquiring early mutations of *TP53* and *KRAS* genes and no mutations of *APC* genes, while in non-inflammatory carcinogenesis of colon, *APC* mutation is the earliest event [33].

Diagnosis of dysplasia is very difficult in UC, since usually, on biopsies taken in active disease, the pathologist identifies significant cellular changes (nuclear polymorphism, hyperchromasia and hypertrophy and sometimes high mitotic activity) related to inflammation and regeneration. But, regenerative changes are usually confined in the base of the crypts, exhibiting unequivocal maturation toward surface and are closely related with the activity of inflammation, while dysplasia lacks maturation and affects, in equal measure, superficial and cryptic epithelium. Also, usually dysplasia associates loss of nuclear polarity, changes in nuclear-cytoplasmic ratio and significant architectural changes. Diagnosis of dysplasia in UC requires architectural abnormalities and cellular alterations beyond regenerative changes [2].

After establishing the diagnosis of unequivocal dysplasia, the pathologist should characterize the nature of the lesion, using microscopic and macroscopic (endoscopic) data: flat dysplasia, adenoma-like dysplasia or dysplasia-associated lesion or mass (DALM) [2]. Furthermore, always it should be kept in mind the fact that patients with UC can have sporadic adenomas with dysplasia, which should be diagnosed like any sporadic adenoma. Usually, diagnosis of dysplasia in UC is formulated using the classical staging of low-grade dysplasia and high-grade dysplasia. Also, there is accepted a diagnosis of "indefinite" for dysplasia in cases with ambiguous cellular anomalies, usually in the vicinity of an ulceration [1, 2, 34]. Low grade dysplasia (LGD) indicates a superficial and cryptic epithelium with hyperchromatic and hypertrophic nuclei that maintain polarization, although with a discrete tendency toward pseudo-stratification. Architectural anomalies are usually mild [2]. High grade dysplasia (HGD) exhibits a more severe architectural distortion and significant cellular atypia with loss of nuclear polarization [2].

Some immunohistochemical markers, such as p53, p21, bcl-2, AMACR (alpha methyl-CoA racemase), can be used to sustain a morphologic diagnosis of dysplasia [1, 29]. Considering that treatment for UC-associated dysplasia is usually colectomy and there is a poor inter- and intraobserver agreement, especially for the diagnosis of LGD, it is mandatory that the diagnosis is confirmed by an independent expert pathologist before any invasive therapy [34–36].

Dysplasia is an indicator of a poor prognosis for the UC patients, with a high risk of evolution toward invasive colorectal adenocarcinoma in the absence of treatment (about 40% for HGD) [37]. LGD has also a high risk of progression toward carcinoma, some recent studies showing that a patient with UC and LGD has a ninefold higher risk for carcinoma than a patient with UC but without dysplasia [1]. One third of patients with LGD, UC and primary sclerosing cholangitis will progress toward more severe neoplastic lesions [38]. About one half of the patients with UC and HGD have already an invasive colorectal carcinoma previously diagnosed [39].

For prognosis reasons, it is very important to know the location of dysplastic lesions, since carcinoma is more frequent in distal segments of the colon in patients with UC [1]. Patients with distal LGD have a higher risk and a shorter period to progression toward HGD than patients with proximal LGD. Also, flat LGD has a higher risk of progression than DALM [1, 40].

3.8. Histologic healing

Histologic mucosal healing can be considered the final goal of treatment in UC, but it is not a current target for treatment because definition is poorly standardized and it is not clear if the risks of additional drug toxicity are acceptable. It is also difficult to obtain, since about one third of the patients with clinical and endoscopical remission still have microscopic inflammation [41].

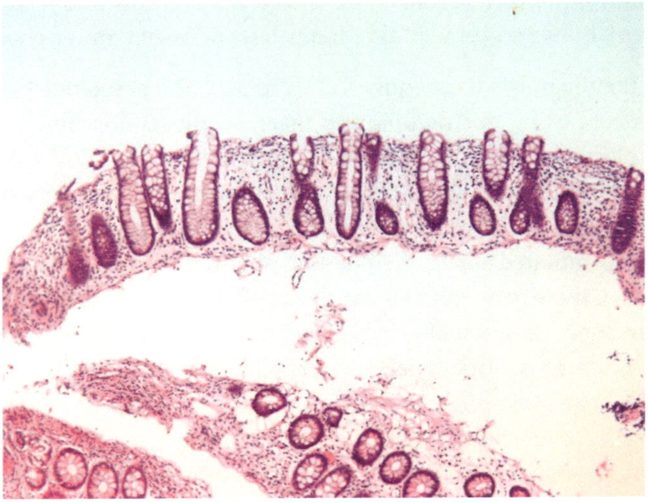

Figure 6. Histologic healing in a patient with repeated flare-ups included in a study for a biological agent. Note some crypts atrophy and irregularities, with normal inflammatory infiltrate and preservation of plasma cell gradient in lamina propria. No neutrophils or eosinophils can be identified (hematoxylin & eosin, 40×).

Histologic healing (**Figure 6**) is usually defined by the remission of inflammatory infiltrate and architectural changes. Some crypt atrophy or reduced crypt density, along with a slight increase of cellularity of lamina propria can persist. Only chronic inflammatory cells are allowed [1]. Complete remission of all lesions can be identified in about one quarter of patients [42]. There are some controversies about the degree of basal plasmacytosis that is acceptable in a patient with histologic healing, since plasma cells are not an indicator of disease activity [25]. Since basal plasmacytosis is, by itself, a poor prognosis marker, we consider that a true histologic healing has no basal plasmacytosis.

Also, it is very important that the diagnosis of histologic healing is formulated only when the pathologist has examined sufficient tissue fragments. Probably, best scenario includes at least two fragments from minimum five sites along the colon, including the rectum and the terminal ileum [1]. This method avoids errors of diagnosis, especially in patients with rectal sparing or skip-lesions, aspects frequently observed after treatment [43].

From all features with predictive value, histologic healing offers the best chance to maintain a sustained remission of the disease [25, 41]. It is, probably, the best indicator of treatment efficacy and the most logical moment for stopping maintenance therapy [44]. Ideally, remission includes clinical, endoscopical and histological resolution, which is called complete remission [45].

4. Conclusions

Histology is an important tool in management of UC patients. Colonic mucosa biopsies are not very difficult to obtain, and routine histologic slides can bring valuable information not only for diagnosis of the disease but also for predicting the patients' outcome.

The highest predictive value for relapse among histologic features is indicated by basal plasmacytosis and histologic healing, while presence of dysplasia indicates the risk for invasive malignancy.

There are still some issues to be clarified concerning histologic scores and their importance in UC management. Also, the term histologic healing needs a better definition until it becomes the ultimate goal of UC treatment.

Acknowledgements

The authors gratefully thank Prof. Dr. Sabina Zurac, Head of Pathology Department in Colentina University Hospital, for her assistance in writing this paper.

Conflict of Interest

The authors declare no conflict of interest.

Authors' contribution

Both authors contribute in equal measure to the conception of the work and have approved the final version of the chapter.

Author details

Cristiana Popp[1*] and Radu Bogdan Mateescu[2]

*Address all correspondence to: brigaela@yahoo.com

1 Colentina University Hospital, Department of Pathology, Bucharest, Romania

2 Colentina University Hospital, Department of Gastroenterology, Carol Davila University of Medicine and Pharmacy, Bucharest, Romania

References

[1] Magro F, Langner C, Driessen A, Ensari A, Geboes K, Mantzaris GJ, Villanacci V, Becheanu G, Borralho Nunes P, Cathomas G, Fries W, Jouret-Mourin A, Mescoli C, de Petris G, Rubio CA, Shepherd NA, Vieth M, Eliakim R. European consensus on the histopathology of inflammatory bowel disease. Journal of Crohn's and Colitis. 2013;**7**(10):827-851. DOI: https://doi.org/10.1016/j.crohns.2013.06.001

[2] DeRoche TC, Xiao SY, Liu X. Histological evaluation in ulcerative colitis. Gastroenterology Report. 2014;**2**(3):178-192. DOI: 10.1093/gastro/gou031

[3] Geboes K. Histopathology of Crohn's disease and ulcerative colitis. In: Satsangi J, Sutherland LR, editors. Inflammatory Bowel Disease. 4th ed. Edinburgh, London, Melbourne: Churchill Livingstone Elsevier; 2003. pp. 255-276

[4] Feakins RM. Inflammatory bowel disease biopsies: Updated British Society of Gastroenterology reporting guidelines. Journal of Clinical Pathology. 2013;**66**:1005-1026. DOI: 10.1136/jclinpath-2013-201885

[5] Samaan MA, Mosli MH, Sandborn WJ, Feagan BG, D'Haens GR, Dubcenco E, Baker KA, Levesque BG. A systematic review of the measurement of endoscopic healing in ulcerative colitis clinical trials: Recommendations and implications for future research. Inflammatory Bowel Diseases. 2014;**20**:1465-1471. DOI: 10.1097/MIB.0000000000000046

[6] Tanaka M, Saito H, Kusumi T, Fukuda S, Shimoyama T, Sasaki Y, Suto K, Munakata A, Kudo H. Spatial distribution and histogenesis of colorectal Paneth cell metaplasia in idiopathic inflammatory bowel disease. Journal of Gastroenterology and Hepatology. 2001;**16**(12):1353-1359

[7] Stange EF, Travis SP, Vermeire S, Reinisch W, Geboes K, Barakauskiene A, Feakins R, Fléjou JF, Herfarth H, Hommes DW, Kupcinskas L, Lakatos PL, Mantzaris GJ, Schreiber S, Villanacci V, Warren BF. European evidence-based consensus on the diagnosis and management of ulcerative colitis: Definitions and diagnosis. Journal of Crohn's and Colitis. 2008;**2**(1):1-23. DOI: 10.1016/j.crohns.2007.11.001

[8] Elphick DA, Mahida YR. Paneth cells: Their role in innate immunity and inflammatory disease. Gut. 2005;**54**(12):1802-1809. DOI: 10.1136/gut.2005.068601

[9] Popp C, Stăniceanu F, Micu G, Nichita L, Cioplea M, Mateescu RB, Voiosu T, Sticlaru L. Evaluation of histologic features with potential prognostic value in ulcerative colitis. Romanian Journal of Internal Medicine. 2014;**52**(4):256-262

[10] Bessissow T, De Hertogh G, Lemmens B, Ferrante M, Bisschops R, Van Steen K, Geboes K, Van Assche G, Vermeire S, Rutgeerts P. Prognostic value of serologic and histologic markers on clinical relapse in ulcerative colitis patients with mucosal healing. The American Journal of Gastroenterology. 2012;**107**(11):1684-1692. DOI: 10.1038/ajg.2012.301

[11] Bitton A, Peppercorn MA, Antonioli DA, Niles JL, Shah S, Bousvaros A, Ransil B, Wild G, Cohen A, Edwardes MD, Stevens AC. Clinical, biological, and histologic parameters as predictors of relapse in ulcerative colitis. Gastroenterology. 2001;**120**(1):13-20

[12] Villanacci V, Antonelli E, Reboldi G, Salemme M, Casella G, Bassotti G. Endoscopic biopsy samples of naive "colitides" patients: Role of basal plasmacytosis. Journal of Crohn's and Colitis. 2014;**8**(11):1438-1443. DOI: 10.1016/j.crohns.2014.05.003

[13] Liverani E, Scaioli E, Digby RJ, Bellanova M, Belluzzi A. How to predict clinical relapse in inflammatory bowel disease patients. World Journal of Gastroenterology. 2016;**22**(3):1017-1033. DOI: 10.3748/wjg.v22.i3.1017

[14] Jauregui-Amezaga A, López-Cerón M, Aceituno M, Jimeno M, Rodríguez de Miguel C, Pinó-Donnay S, Zabalza M, Sans M, Ricart E, Ordás I, González-Suárez B, Cuatrecasas M, Llach J, Panés J, Pellise M. Accuracy of advanced endoscopy and fecal calprotectin for prediction of relapse in ulcerative colitis: A prospective study. Inflammatory Bowel Diseases. 2014;**20**:1187-1193. DOI: 10.1097/MIB.0000000000000069

[15] Al-Haddad S, Riddell RH. The role of eosinophils in inflammatory bowel disease. Gut. 2005;**54**:1674-1675. DOI: 10.1136/gut.2005.072595

[16] Lampinen M, Rönnblom A, Amin K, Kristjansson G, Rorsman F, Sangfelt P, Säfsten B, Wagner M, Wanders A, Winqvist O, Carlson M. Eosinophil granulocytes are activated during the remission phase of ulcerative colitis. Gut. 2005;**54**:1714-1720. DOI: 10.1136/gut.2005.066423

[17] Zezos P, Patsiaoura K, Nakos A, Mpoumponaris A, Vassiliadis T, Giouleme O, Pitiakoudis M, Kouklakis G, Evgenidis N. Severe eosinophilic infiltration in colonic biopsies predicts patients with ulcerative colitis not responding to medical therapy. Colorectal Disease. 2014;**16**(12):O420-O430. DOI: 10.1111/codi.12725

[18] Azad S, Sood N, Sood A. Biological and histological parameters as predictors of relapse in ulcerative colitis: A prospective study. Saudi Journal of Gastroenterology: Official Journal of the Saudi Gastroenterology Association. 2011;**17**(3):194-198. DOI: 10.4103/1319-3767.80383

[19] Melson JE, Giusto D, Kwasny M, Eichenseer P, Jakate S, Keshavarzian A. Histopathology predictors of medically refractory ulcerative colitis. Diseases of the Colon and Rectum. 2010;**53**:1280-1286. DOI: 10.1007/DCR.0b013e3181e751df

[20] Geboes K, Riddell R, Ost A, Jensfelt B, Persson T, Löfberg R. A reproducible grading scale for histological assessment of inflammation in ulcerative colitis. Gut. 2000;**47**:404-409. DOI: 10.1136/gut.47.3.404

[21] Zenlea T, Yee EU, Rosenberg L, Boyle M, Nanda KS, Wolf JL, Falchuk KR, Cheifetz AS, Goldsmith JD, Moss AC. Histology grade is independently associated with relapse risk in patients with ulcerative colitis in clinical remission: A prospective study. The American Journal of Gastroenterology. 2016;**111**(5):685-690. DOI: 10.1038/ajg.2016.50

[22] Jauregui-Amezaga A, Geerits A, Das Y, Lemmens B, Sagaert X, Bessissow T, Lobatón T, Ferrante M, Van Assche G, Bisschops R, Geboes K, De Hertogh G, Vermeire S. A simplified Geboes score for ulcerative colitis. Journal of Crohn's & Colitis. 2017;**11**(3):305-313. DOI: 10.1093/ecco-jcc/jjw154

[23] Marchal-Bressenot A, Salleron J, Boulagnon-Rombi C, Bastien C, Cahn V, Cadiot G, Diebold MD, Danese S, Reinisch W, Schreiber S, Travis S, Peyrin-Biroulet L. Development and validation of the Nancy histological index for UC. Gut. 2017;**66**(1):43-49. DOI: 10.1136/gutjnl-2015-310187

[24] Siegel CA, Whitman CB, Spiegel BM, Feagan B, Sands B, Loftus EV Jr, Panaccione R, D'Haens G, Bernstein CN, Gearry R, Ng SC, Mantzaris GJ, Sartor B, Silverberg MS, Riddell R, Koutroubakis IE, O'Morain C, Lakatos PL, McGovern DP, Halfvarson J, Reinisch W, Rogler G, Kruis W, Tysk C, Schreiber S, Danese S, Sandborn W, Griffiths A, Moum B, Gasche C, Pallone F, Travis S, Panes J, Colombel JF, Hanauer S, Peyrin-Biroulet L. Development of an index to define overall disease severity in IBD. Gut. 2016;**10**:25. DOI: 10.1136/gutjnl-2016-312648

[25] Villanacci V, Antonelli E, Lanzarotto F, Bozzola A, Cadei M, Bassotti G. Usefulness of different pathological scores to assess healing of the mucosa in inflammatory bowel diseases: A real life study. Scientific Reports. 2017;**7**:6839. DOI: 10.1038/s41598-017-07338-x

[26] Walsh AJ, Bryant RV, Travis SP. Current best practice for disease activity assessment in IBD. Nature Reviews. Gastroenterology & Hepatology. 2016;**13**(10):567-579. DOI: 10.1038/nrgastro.2016.128

[27] Feagan BG, Greenberg GR, Wild G, Fedorak RN, Paré P, McDonald JW, Dubé R, Cohen A, Steinhart AH, Landau S, Aguzzi RA, Fox IH, Vandervoort MK. Treatment of ulcerative colitis with a humanized antibody to the α4β7 integrin. The New England Journal of Medicine. 2005;**352**(24):2499-2507. DOI: 10.1056/NEJMoa042982

[28] Feagins LA, Melton SD, Iqbal R, Dunbar KB, Spechler SJ. Clinical implications of histologic abnormalities in colonic biopsy specimens from patients with ulcerative colitis in clinical remission. Inflammatory Bowel Diseases. 2013;**19**:1477-1482. DOI: 10.1097/MIB.0b013e318281f4ae

[29] Popp C, Nichita L, Voiosu T, et al. Expression profile of p53 and p21 in large bowel mucosa as biomarkers of inflammatory-related carcinogenesis in ulcerative colitis. Disease Markers. 2016;**2016**:3625279. DOI: 10.1155/2016/3625279

[30] Longman R, Warren B. Is the colonic reparative cell lineage yet to be discovered? Gut. 2000;**47**(2):307-308. DOI: 10.1136/gut.47.2.307

[31] Imai T, Fukuta K, Hasumura M, Cho YM, Ota Y, Takami S, Nakagama H, Hirose M. Significance of inflammation-associated regenerative mucosa characterized by Paneth cell metaplasia and beta-catenin accumulation for the onset of colorectal carcinogenesis in rats initiated with 1,2-dimethylhydrazine. Carcinogenesis. 2007;**28**:2199-2206. DOI: 10.1093/carcin/bgm118

[32] Cunliffe R, Rose F, Keyte J, Abberley L, Chan W, Mahida Y. Human defensin 5 is stored in precursor form in normal Paneth cells and is expressed by some villous epithelial cells and by metaplastic Paneth cells in the colon in inflammatory bowel disease. Gut. 2001;**48**(2):176-185. DOI: 10.1136/gut.48.2.176

[33] Humphries A, Jawad N, Ignjatovic N, East J, Leedham S. Carcinogenesis in ulcerative colitis. In: Shennak M, editor. Ulcerative Colitis from Genetics to Complications. InTech; 2012. DOI: 10.5772/25306

[34] Riddell RH, Goldman H, Ransohoff DF, Appelman HD, Fenoglio CM, Haggitt RC, Hren C, Correa P, Hamilton SR, Morson BC, Sommers SC, Yardley JH. Dysplasia in inflammatory bowel disease: Standardized classification with provisional clinical application. Human Pathology. 1983;**14**(11):931-968. DOI: 10.1016/S0046-8177(83)80175-0

[35] Eaden J, Abrams K, McKay H, Denley H, Mayberry J. Inter-observer variation between general and specialist gastrointestinal pathologists when grading dysplasia in ulcerative colitis. The Journal of Pathology. 2001;**194**:152-157. DOI: 10.1002/path.876

[36] Odze RD, Goldblum J, Noffsinger A, Alsaigh N, Rybicki LA, Fogt F. Interobserver variability in the diagnosis of ulcerative colitis-associated dysplasia by telepathology. Modern Pathology. 2002;**15**:379-386. DOI: 10.1038/modpathol.3880534

[37] Rutter MD, Saunders BP, Wilkinson KH, Rumbles S, Schofield G, Kamm MA, Williams CB, Price AB, Talbot IC, Forbes A. Thirty-year analysis of a colonoscopic surveillance program for neoplasia in ulcerative colitis. Gastroenterology. 2006;**130**:1030-1038. DOI: 10.1053/j.gastro.2005.12.035

[38] Venkatesh PG, Jegadeesan R, Gutierrez NG, Sanaka MR, Navaneethan U. Natural history of low grade dysplasia in patients with primary sclerosing cholangitis and ulcerative colitis. Journal of Crohn's and Colitis. 2013;**7**(12):968-973. DOI: 10.1016/j.crohns.2013.02.002

[39] Farraye F, Odze R, Eaden J, Itzkowitz SAGA. Technical review on the diagnosis and management of colorectal neoplasia in inflammatory bowel disease. Gastroenterology. 2010;**138**(2):738-745. DOI: 10.1053/j.gastro.2009.12.037

[40] Goldstone R, Itzkowitz S, Harpaz N, Ullman T. Progression of low-grade dysplasia in ulcerative colitis: Effect of colonic location. Gastrointestinal Endoscopy. 2011;**74**:1087-1093. DOI: 10.1016/j.gie.2011.06.028

[41] Park S, Abdi T, Gentry M, Laine L. Histological disease activity as a predictor of clinical relapse among patients with ulcerative colitis: Systematic review and meta-analysis. The American Journal of Gastroenterology. 2016;**111**:1692-1701. DOI: 10.1038/ajg.2016.418

[42] Levine TS, Tzardi M, Mitchell S, Sowter C, Price AB. Diagnostic difficulty arising from rectal recovery in ulcerative colitis. Journal of Clinical Pathology. 1996;**49**(4):319-323

[43] Villanacci V, Antonelli E, Geboes K, Casella G, Bassotti G. Histological healing in inflammatory bowel disease: A still unfulfilled promise. World Journal of Gastroenterology. 2013;**19**(7):968-978. DOI: 10.3748/wjg.v19.i7.968

[44] Guardiola J, Arajol C, Armuzzi A. Is histologic remission in ulcerative colitis ready for prime time? Digestive and Liver Disease. 2017;**49**(12):1334-1335. DOI: 10.1016/j.dld.2017.09.130

[45] Bryant RV, Winer S, Travis SP, Riddell RH. Systematic review: Histological remission in inflammatory bowel disease. Is 'complete' remission the new treatment paradigm? An IOIBD initiative. Journal of Crohn's and Colitis. 2014;**8**(12):1582-1597. DOI: 10.1016/j.crohns.2014.08.011

Section 3

Clinical Menifestation of Inflammatory Bowel Disease

Chapter 3

Neurological Manifestations of Inflammatory Bowel Disease

Julio Plata-Bello and Silvia Acosta-López

Additional information is available at the end of the chapter

http://dx.doi.org/10.5772/intechopen.73017

Abstract

The inflammatory bowel disease (IBD) is associated with different neurological and psychiatric disorders, which are integrated among the extra-intestinal manifestation of this disease. The physiopathology of neurological manifestations of IBD varies among the different kind of complications. The origin and the significance of these manifestations must be understood by clinicians who manage IBD patients. Some of them are related to therapeutic agents. The present chapter consists of a review of the most prevalent neurological and psychiatric disorders associated with IBD. The physiopathology of those entities will also be discussed, as well as the appropriate management for their prevention and treatment.

Keywords: neurological disorders, psychiatric disorders, thrombosis, demyelination, peripheral neuropathy, extra-intestinal manifestations

1. Introduction

Inflammatory bowel disease (IBD) is a chronic disease of the gastrointestinal tract with an unknown etiology, which alternates between periods of symptoms relapse and remission [1, 2]. IBD involves various entities. Crohn's disease (CD) and ulcerative colitis (UC) are the most common, but other inflammatory conditions of the gastrointestinal tract are also included under this term, such as the indeterminate colitis, microscopic colitis and pouchitis [3]. In the present chapter, only CD and UC are discussed.

The incidence of IBD is different depending on its two main forms. CD is diagnosed in 0.5–10.6 patients/100,000 inhabitants/year, while the global incidence of UC is estimated at 0.9–24.3 patients/100,000 inhabitants/year. There is some evidence about the increase of these incidence figures in the past 10 years [2]. On the other hand, the prevalence of CD in European countries ranges from 1.5 to 213 cases per 100,000 people and the prevalence of UC ranges from 2.4 to 294 cases per 100,000 people [2].

IBD consists of an inflammation of the bowel, with different extension and histological features between CD and UC. However, this disease does not only involve the gastrointestinal tract, but there is also a long list of extraintestinal manifestations that can emerge prior to or during the disease. The most frequent ones are those involving the skin (dermatological), the joints (rheumatological), the eyes (ophthalmological), the liver and/or the biliary tract and the genitourinary area (gynecological and/or urological). The prevalence of at least one extraintestinal manifestation varies from 6.2 to 46.6% [4].

Neurological manifestations of IBD are unusual, but they are potentially harmful, leading to severe and irreversible consequences if they are not detected and managed early and properly. The prevalence of neurological manifestations has not been appropriately established, but some authors have reported a prevalence of 20–30%, although there is a general belief that subclinical or unrecognized neurological impairment may be present in IBD patients [4–6].

The aim of the present chapter is to briefly review the main neurological manifestations associated with IBD, with a special focus on their physiopathological mechanisms.

2. General pathophysiological considerations of IBD and its neurological manifestations

Although a specific etiological agent in the development of IBD has not been established, it is widely accepted that some scenarios may be associated with the development of this disease [4]:

- An inflammatory reaction to a persistent bowel infection.
- The presence of defects in the barrier of the intestinal mucosa to act against certain antigens.
- The presence of disturbances in the immune response to certain antigens.

In this regard, a dysfunction of the immune system and a chronic inflammatory response appear both in the context of a specific environmental situation and in a genetically predisposed patient [1]. However, bearing in mind the physiopathology of neurological manifestations, there are different mechanisms that may specifically be involved in their development [4]:

- Malabsorption and secondary deficit of vitamins (mainly vitamin B12), which are essential for myelin maintenance and regeneration [7].
- Hypercoagulability state, related to a chronic inflammatory response that may lead to ischemic events.
- Formation of metabolic toxic agents in the damaged bowel.
- Immunological disturbances that may lead to autoimmune response against glial-neural components.
- Opportunistic infections secondary to the impairment of the immune system or because of the treatment for IBD.

http://dx.doi.org/10.5772/intechopen.73017

These mechanisms can lead to neurological damage acting individually or in combination. The identification of the leading mechanism is essential to prevent greater neurological damage. Unfortunately, in many cases, it is not possible to identify the main pathological factor.

Nevertheless, disease-related mechanisms are not the only ones that need to be considered to understand the origin of neurological manifestations. The pharmacological agents usually used in IBD may also lead to the development of such manifestations. The appropriate selection of a therapeutic agent depends on the subtype of disease (CD or UC), location and phenotype of the disease [8].

Some of these treatments try to prevent new relapses of the disease, whereas others try to control the symptoms during a relapse. The vast majority of these therapeutic agents can produce neurological manifestations as an adverse effect (**Table 1**), thus clinicians always have to consider the possibility that neurological manifestations in IBD patients may have a pharmacological rather than a primary IBD-related origin.

Drug category		**High frequency (>1 case per 100 patients)**	**Low frequency (>1 case per 1000 patients)**	**Rare (>1 case per 10,000 patients)**	**Unknown frequency**
Steroids				Seizures. Development or worsening of psychiatric disorders (euphoria, mood and personality changes, depression and psychosis)	Dizziness, headache, insomnia
5-Aminosalicilates				Headache, dizziness and peripheral neuropathy	
Antibiotics	Metronidazole	Seizures, peripheral neuropathy. Others: dizziness, ataxia, incoordination, confusion, irritability depression, weakness, insomnia and encephalopathy			
	Ciprofloxacin		Headache, dizziness, sleep disorders, taste disorders, motor hyperactivity	Sensitive disturbances, tremor, seizures, migraine, incoordination, olfactory disorders, confusion, anxiety, depression, psychotic reactions	Peripheral neuropathy
Ciclosporin A		Tremor, headache, seizures, paresthesia	Encephalopathy, confusion, disorientation, decrease level consciousness, anxiety, insomnia, visual disturbances, cortical blindness, comma, paresia and ataxia	Motor polyneuropathy, optic nerve edema	Migraine

Methotrexate		Paresthesia	Motor weakness, encephalopathy, seizures and headache	Mood disorders and cognitive disturbances. Motor weakness, aphasia, cranial nerve disturbances	Intracranial hypertension, neurotoxicity, arachnoiditis, paraplegia, astonishment, ataxia, dementia, dizziness
Thiopurines	Azathioprine			Myasthenic crisis, paresia, polyneuritis	Progressive multifocal leucoencephalopathy when other immunosuppressors are combined
	6-Mercaptopurine	Not reported			
Anti-TNF	Infliximab	Headache, dizziness	Depression, confusion, amnesia, anxiety apathy, drowsiness. Demyelinating disease exacerbation		
	Adalimumab	Mood changes (depression), anxiety, insomnia. Headache, paresthesias, migraine, radicular compression	Cerebrovascular accident, tremor, neuropathy	Multiple sclerosis and other myelinating disorders (optic neuritis and Guillain-Barré syndrome)	
	Certolizumab pegol			Demyelinating disease, including multiple sclerosis (onset or exacerbation). Seizures, peripheral neuropathy	
	Golimumab	Dizziness, headache, paresthesias. Depression, insomnia	Instability	Multiple sclerosis and other demyelinating diseases, dysgeusia	
Vedolizumab		Headache, paresthesia			
Ustekinumab		Dizziness, headache	Depression. Facial palsy		

Table 1. IBD treatment-related neurological complications with categorization of their frequency.

3. Venous and arterial thrombotic and thromboembolic manifestations

Thromboembolic events are common in the context of IBD, secondary to the hypercoagulability state that exists in this disease. This hypercoagulability is associated with an increase of coagulation-associated factors and thrombin levels, as well as fibrin formation; a decrease of natural anticoagulant factors; a decrease in fibrinolytic activity; the presence of endothelial anomalies; and an increase in the count and activity of platelets [9].

Overall, the incidence of thrombotic complications is 1.2–7.5% in clinical studies, but this can rise to 39% when post-mortem studies are considered [10, 11]. Both arterial and venous system may be affected, but deep venous thrombosis and pulmonary thromboembolism are the most common thromboembolic complications in IBD [10–13].

Intracranial thromboembolic events are much less frequent. Cerebral venous thrombosis is more common in CU than in CD, and this may involve superficial or deep cerebral venous systems or even some of the brain venous sinus [11, 14]. The risk of thrombotic or thromboembolic complications in the brain is clearly associated with the activity of the disease. During these periods, IBD patients have a higher risk of cerebral thromboembolic complications than the normal population [9, 10]. These events are rarely reported during periods of non-activity of the disease [9, 10], although some authors have described a higher incidence of thromboembolic events in IBD patients than in healthy controls not only during a relapse of the disease but also during remission periods [15]. Larger cohort and case-control studies are needed to confirm this finding, because if IBD patients suffer more thromboembolic events even during remission periods, anticoagulant therapies might be routinely indicated.

In any case, the increase of thromboembolic events during relapses is clearly related to the inflammatory response whose effect in the coagulation and platelet system has been described above. Nevertheless, the use of steroids, dehydration, the increase of homocysteine and infections (all of which are associated with relapsing periods) may also contribute to the development of thrombotic complications [10–13, 16]. Furthermore, the presence of mutations in Leiden factor V in IBD patients leads to a higher incidence of thrombotic events [17].

Therefore, bearing in mind the high risk of thromboembolic events in IBD patients, mostly during relapses [18, 19], it is essential to rapidly initiate a primary prophylaxis, with an early mobilization, a correct rehydration and vitamin reposition, as well as the use of prophylactic anticoagulants (mainly low molecular weight heparins). All of these measures are proven to be useful in the prevention of venous thromboembolic events [20].

On the other hand, IBD patients also seem to present a higher incidence of arterial thromboembolic events. Indeed, many studies have reported an association between cardiovascular events and other chronic inflammatory diseases, like rheumatoid arthritis, lupus or psoriasis [21–23]. Active IBD is also associated with a higher risk of cardiovascular events (spontaneous or after surgical/invasive procedures), especially in young female patients [9].

When arterial thromboembolic events occur in the brain, they can be classified as ischemic stroke. Although the literature agrees about the high risk of thromboembolic events in IBD patients, the increase in the incidence of ischemic stroke in IBD patients is a matter of debate [9]. In this regard, Huang et al. [24], in a large retrospective cohort study, analyzed the risk of ischemic stroke in IBD patients of a Taiwanese population. Although the studied groups were not completely comparable in demographical and comorbidity features, the authors reported a higher prevalence of ischemic stroke in IBD patients (mainly in CD patients) than the general population (hazard ratios for UC and CD were 1.01 [95% confidence interval = 0.84–1.21] and 1.15 [95% confidence interval = 1.04–1.28], respectively) [24]. Similar results were reported in a Danish population-based setting (also with a mismatch in comorbidity distribution), showing a relative risk (RR) of 1.15 of suffering ischemic stroke in an IBD population (95% confidence interval 1.04–1.27) of suffering ischemic stroke in an IBD population [25]. Therefore, there is weak evidence of the higher incidence of ischemic stroke in IBD populations. In any case, it seems to be of the utmost importance to manage cardiovascular risk factors in IBD patients [9]. Their combination with the pro-thrombotic situation that may be present in any phase of IBD can play a major role in the development of brain ischemic complications, which are associated with a high level of dependence and an important worsening of quality of life.

However, vascular events may not be only associated with pro-thrombotic conditions. Vasculitis may also contribute to the presence of neurological manifestations. Bearing this in mind, systemic vasculitis is also considered an extra-intestinal manifestation of IBD. Wegener's granulomatosis, Takayasu arteritis, medial temporal arteritis and Cogan's syndrome (among others) have been reported in combination with IBD [4, 26]. For example, Takayasu arteritis is associated with IBD in 9.6% of cases [27], and this frequency seems to be higher in CD patients (9%) [28] than in UC (6.4%) [29]. The pathogenesis of vasculitis associated with IBD is mediated by immune complex deposits and cytotoxic lymphocytes [30]. The vasculitis of IBD patients involves medium and large caliber vessels and may lead to brain ischemic events [4], and some of them can directly affect the central nervous system (CNS) [31]. The global frequency of vasculitis associated with IBD is unknown, but it has been reported that such cases of vasculitis involving the CNS are rare [31]. Furthermore, this manifestation seems to be independent of the activity of the disease in the gastrointestinal tract [30, 32]. A correct diagnosis of CNS vasculitis is essential, because it allows the initiation of the appropriate treatment and the prevention of significant neurological impairment. Thus, when IBD patients present any CNS vascular event, vasculitis must be considered as a possible diagnosis and it has to be appropriately ruled out.

4. Demyelinating diseases

The association of demyelinating diseases has been proposed since the early 1980s. Rang et al. described a higher prevalence of multiple sclerosis (MS) than expected in UC patients [33]. Subsequently, this finding has been confirmed by many reports, but not only for UC but also for CD [34–36]. For instance, Gupta et al. described an increased risk of optic neuritis and other forms of MS in CD (odds ratio = 1.54) and UC (odds ratio = 1.75) [35]. In the same line, a recent meta-analysis concluded that IBD patients present a higher risk of suffering from concomitant MS and vice versa (i.e. MS patients have a higher risk of suffering from associated IBD) [36]. These authors found an increased risk of 50% [36].

However, some authors have proposed that the development of demyelinating diseases in IBD patients is more related to the use of anti-TNFα drugs [37]. In this regard, the Spanish registry of autoimmune adverse events of biological agents (BIOGEAS Project) reported 12 cases of MS and 25 cases of optic neuritis in IBD patients treated with anti-TNFα [38]. Furthermore, this phenomenon is not exclusive to IBD patients. Arthritis patients treated with anti-TNFα agents may develop MS or demyelinating lesions, with a partial or complete resolution of neurological symptoms after discontinuing the medication [39]. An increased number of new white matter lesions and new relapses have also been reported in MS patients treated with infliximab [40]. On the other hand, the use of Natalizumab, a monoclonal antibody against alfa4-integrin used in some cases of IBD, is associated with progressive multifocal leukoencephalopathy (PML). This disease appears after a reactivation of the JC virus infection, and the use of Natalizumab is clearly associated with this reactivation. PML is associated with a bad prognosis with a mortality rate at 6 months above 60% [37].

Apart from demyelinating diseases associated with IBD, there is strong evidence of a higher prevalence of white matter lesions in neurologically asymptomatic IBD patients than in healthy subjects [5, 41]. Although these lesions are usually asymptomatic, their number and volume tend to increase with age (mostly in CU patients) [41]. In any case, whenever these lesions become symptomatic, their association with other CNS complications (e.g. cerebrovascular complications) has to be identified.

Therefore, in spite of the plausible relationship between MS and IBD, the presence of white matter lesions is not evidence of the coexistence of both diseases. In fact, most of these lesions have no clinical relevance and their presence in IBD patients should not be used to infer active CNS disease [42]. Further research is needed about the origin of these lesions and their neurological and cognitive consequences in IBD patients.

5. Epilepsy

The relationship between epilepsy and IBD is uncertain. Lossos et al. reported a prevalence of 1.9% in a cohort of 638 IBD patients, although the majority of these patients had a structural and/or metabolic cause that may lead to epileptic seizures [32]. Other authors have reported an improvement of seizures in CD patients after treatment initiation, suggesting that immunological mechanisms may be associated with the development of this disorder [43]. This finding might also be supported by some case reports [44].

However, the most plausible explanation for the development of epileptic seizures in IBD patients is that other CNS complications (e.g. thromboembolic events or unspecific white matter lesions) or other systemic complications (e.g. dehydration, low levels of magnesium, etc.) may facilitate its development [45, 46]. Because of the above, a correct therapeutic management may help to resolve and/or prevent this condition.

6. Peripheral neuropathy

Peripheral neuropathy (PN) is one of the most common neurological complications in IBD patients [32, 43, 47]. Many factors have been associated with the development of PN, such as extraintestinal inflammation, immunological phenomena, nutritional disturbances (e.g. malabsorption-related vitamin deficit) and adverse effects of IBD therapeutic agents (e.g. metronidazole or anti-TNF agents) [48–50]. Whenever these causes are ruled out, the frequency of PN in IBD patients varies from 0 to 39% [51].

IBD-associated PN may be associated with axonal damage or demyelination and it may have an acute or chronic presentation [47, 51]. Cases of mononeuropathy, plexopathies, multiple mononeuritis, compressive neuropathies and cranial neuropathies have also been reported [50]. Bearing this in mind, IBD-related PNs present great clinical variability, although there is a certain dominance of non-demyelinating vs. myelinating forms [48].

Demyelinating forms have a better prognosis than non-demyelinating forms, because they have a more favorable response to immunotherapy. This situation may be related to the role that T lymphocytes seem to play in demyelinating IBD-associated PNs. On the other hand, the relationship between axonal PNs and immunological disturbances is less clear [47, 48].

7. Psychiatric disorders

IBD patients show a high prevalence of psychiatric disorders, with depression and anxiety as the main diagnosis [1, 52, 53]. The prevalence of depression in IBD patients varies from 15 to 30%, but the frequency of anxiety rises to 80%, mainly associated with the relapses of the disease [54, 55]. There is no overall difference in the frequency of psychiatric disorders between UC and CD [52].

Several factors have been associated with IBD-related depression: female gender, active intestinal disease, the presence of fistulas or perianal disease, use of biological treatments and the necessity of surgery because of IBD [55]. On the other hand, IBD patients with IBD seem to present more aggressive phenotypes of the disease, with more relapses and shorter periods of remission [52]. In any case, the prevalence of depression or anxiety is even higher when other psychiatric conditions coexist [1, 52, 53].

Anyway, depression and anxiety are not the only IBD- associated psychiatric disorders. The Manitoba IBD Cohort Study reported a higher prevalence in IBD patients than in general population of panic and obsessive-compulsive disorders [56]. Controversy exists around bipolar disorder. On the one hand, the Manitoba IBD Cohort Study reported a lower prevalence of bipolar disorder in IBD than in the general population. On the other hand, Eaton et al. (2010) reported a higher frequency of this psychiatric condition in IBD patients, more specifically in CD patients [57].

However, it is widely accepted that there is an infra-diagnosis and infra-treatment of psychiatric disorders, with no systematic screening established in clinical guidelines. There is a strong evidence of the presence of a bidirectional relationship between the degree of inflammation in the gastrointestinal tract and the development of depression. This can be explained by the brain-gut axis hypothesis. The brain and the gut are communicated by the autonomic nervous system (sympathetic and parasympathetic systems). The vagus nerve (the main parasympathetic afferent) transmits information to the CNS about luminal osmolarity, carbohydrate levels, mechanical distortion of the mucosa and the presence of bacterial or cytostatic drugs. On the other hand, sympathetic afferents transmit visceral pain [58].

Information sent by the gastrointestinal system reaches the medulla (nucleus tractus solitarius) and travels upstream until it reaches the paraventricular nucleus where it finally modulates the hypothalamic–pituitary–adrenal (HPA) axis [59].

Some authors proposed that an impairment in the gut-brain axis can be induced by stress. In this regard, stressful situations lead to a vagal inhibition and an overactivation of the sympathetic system. These conditions associated with other CNS-mediated responses involving the modulation of the immune system and the HPA axis may be associated with the appearance of a gastrointestinal immunoinflammatory response [58, 60]. For instance, during depression, an elevation of alpha-TNF, IL-1, reactive C protein and haptoglobin and a decrease of IL-10, TGF-B, albumin and transferrin are observed [61].

Therefore, there is a notable association between IBD and psychiatric disorders. New studies are necessary to elucidate in which cases the psychiatric condition is the cause or the consequence of IBD. This may help to understand pathophysiological aspects of IBD that are still unknown and ultimately may allow better management of the disease.

8. Conclusion

IBD patients may suffer from different neurological manifestations during their disease. The pathophysiological mechanisms involved in these complications are variable and, in many cases, they are still unrecognized. Anyway, clinicians must stay focused on the early identification of IBD neurological complications and to rapidly establish the appropriate management to prevent further impairment.

Author details

Julio Plata-Bello[1]* and Silvia Acosta-López[2]

*Address all correspondence to: jplata5@hotmail.com

1 Department of Neurosurgery, Hospital Universitario de Canarias, S/C de Tenerife, Spain

2 Department of Gastroenterology and Hepatology, Hospital Universitario Nuestra Señora de La Candelaria, S/C de Tenerife, Spain

References

[1] Abautret-Daly Á, Dempsey E, Parra-Blanco A, Medina C, Harkin A. Gut–brain actions underlying comorbid anxiety and depression associated with inflammatory bowel disease. Acta Neuropsychiatrica. 2017;**8**:1-22

[2] Burisch J, Jess T, Martinato M, Lakatos PL. The burden of inflammatory bowel disease in Europe. Journal of Crohn's and Colitis. 2013;**7**(4):322-337

[3] Montoro MA, García Pagán JC. Enfermedad inflamatoria intestinal. Enfermedad de Crohn. In: Gastroenterología y Hepatología Problemas comunes en la práctica clínica. 2nd ed. Madrid: Jarpyo Editores; 2012. pp. 443-458

[4] Bermejo PE, Burgos A. Complicaciones neurológicas de la enfermedad inflamatoria intestinal. Medicina Clínica (Barcelona). 2008;**130**(17):666-675

[5] Geissler A, Andus T, Roth M, Kullmann F, Caesar I, Held P, et al. Focal white-matter lesions in brain of patients with inflammatory bowel disease. Lancet (London, England). 1995 Apr;**345**(8954):897-898

[6] Lindgren S, Lilja B, Rosén I, Sundkvist G. Disturbed autonomic nerve function in patients with Crohn's disease. Scandinavian Journal of Gastroenterology. 1991 Apr;**26**(4): 361-366

[7] Mariño Suárez JE, Monedero Recuero I, Peláez Laguno C. Deficiencia de vitamina B12 y tratamiento por vía oral. Una opción tan eficaz como (todavía) poco utilizada. Atención Primaria. 2003;**32**(6):382-387

[8] Bernstein CN, Eliakim A, Fedail S, Fried M, Gearry R, Goh K-L, et al. Update. Journal of Clinical Gastroenterology. August 2015;**50**(10):803-818

[9] Zezos P, Kouklakis G, Saibil F. Inflammatory bowel disease and thromboembolism. World Journal of Gastroenterology. 2014;**20**(38):13863-13878

[10] Benarroch HS, Acosta AV. Complicaciones vasculares asociadas a la enfermedad inflamatoria intestinal. Anales de Medicina Interna. 2003;**20**:81-84

[11] Ashrafi MR, Hosseini F, Alizadeh H. Case report pseudotumor cerebri in a case of ulcerative colitis with sagittal sinus thrombosis case presentation. Iranian Journal of Pediatrics. 2013;**23**(1):109-112

[12] Lloyd-Still JD, Tomasi L. Neurovascular and thromboembolic complications of inflammatory bowel disease in childhood. Journal of Pediatric Gastroenterology and Nutrition. 1989 Nov;**9**(4):461-466

[13] Papa A, Gerardi V, Marzo M, Felice C, Rapaccini GL, Gasbarrini A. Venous thromboembolism in patients with inflammatory bowel disease: Focus on prevention and treatment. World Journal of Gastroenterology. 2014;**20**(12):3173-3179

[14] Cho Y, Chae MK, Cha JM, Il LJ, Joo KR, Shin HP, et al. Cerebral venous thrombosis in a patient with Crohn's disease. Intestinal Research. 2016;**14**(1):96-101

[15] Grainge MJ, West J, Card TR. Venous thromboembolism during active disease and remission in inflammatory bowel disease: A cohort study. Lancet. 2010;**375**(9715):657-663

[16] Twig G, Zandman-Goddard G, Szyper-Kravitz M, Shoenfeld Y. Systemic thromboembolism in inflammatory bowel disease: Mechanisms and clinical applications. Annals of the New York Academy of Sciences. 2005 Jun;**1051**:166-173

[17] Liebman HA, Kashani N, Sutherland D, McGehee W, Kam AL. The factor V Leiden mutation increases the risk of venous thrombosis in patients with inflammatory bowel disease. Gastroenterology. 1998 Oct;**115**(4):830-834

[18] Van Assche G, Dignass A, Reinisch W, van der Woude CJ, Sturm A, De Vos M, et al. The second European evidence-based consensus on the diagnosis and management of Crohn's disease: Special situations. Journal of Crohn's & Colitis. 2010 Feb;**4**(1):63-101

[19] Van Assche G, Dignass A, Bokemeyer B, Danese S, Gionchetti P, Moser G, et al. Second European evidence-based consensus on the diagnosis and management of ulcerative colitis part 3: Special situations. Journal of Crohn's & Colitis. 2013 Feb;**7**(1):1-33

[20] Dentali F, Douketis JD, Gianni M, Lim W, Crowther MA. Meta-analysis: Anticoagulant prophylaxis to prevent symptomatic venous thromboembolism in hospitalized medical patients. Annals of Internal Medicine. 2007 Feb;**146**(4):278-288

[21] Ahlehoff O, Gislason GH, Charlot M, Jørgensen CH, Lindhardsen J, Olesen JB, et al. Psoriasis is associated with clinically significant cardiovascular risk: A Danish nationwide cohort study. Journal of Internal Medicine. 2011 Aug;**270**(2):147-157

[22] Meune C, Touzé E, Trinquart L, Allanore Y. Trends in cardiovascular mortality in patients with rheumatoid arthritis over 50 years: A systematic review and meta-analysis of cohort studies. Rheumatology (Oxford, England). 2009 Oct;**48**(10):1309-1313

[23] Svenungsson E, Jensen-Urstad K, Heimbürger M, Silveira A, Hamsten A, de Faire U, et al. Risk factors for cardiovascular disease in systemic lupus erythematosus. Circulation. 2001 Oct;**104**(16):1887-1893

[24] Huang WS, Tseng CH, Chen PC, Tsai CH, Lin CL, Sung FC, et al. Inflammatory bowel diseases increase future ischemic stroke risk: A Taiwanese population-based retrospective cohort study. European Journal of Internal Medicine. 2014;**25**(6):561-565

[25] Kristensen SL, Ahlehoff O, Lindhardsen J, Erichsen R, Jensen GV, Torp-Pedersen C, et al. Disease activity in inflammatory bowel disease is associated with increased risk of myocardial infarction, stroke and cardiovascular death—A Danish nationwide cohort study. PLoS One. 2013;**8**(2):e56944

[26] Sy A, Khalidi N, Dehghan N, Barra L, Carette S, Cuthbertson D, et al. Vasculitis in patients with inflammatory bowel diseases: A study of 32 patients and systematic review of the literature. Seminars in Arthritis and Rheumatism. 2016 Feb;**45**(4):475-482

[27] Akiyama S, Fujii T, Matsuoka K, Yusuke E, Negi M, Takenaka K, et al. Endoscopic features and genetic background of inflammatory bowel disease complicated with Takayasu arteritis. Journal of Gastroenterology and Hepatology. 2017 May;**32**(5):1011-1017

[28] Reny J-L, Paul J-F, Lefèbvre C, Champion K, Emmerich J, Blétry O, et al. Association of Takayasu's arteritis and Crohn's disease. Results of a study on 44 Takayasu patients and review of the literature. Annales de Medecine Interne. 2003 Mar;**154**(2):85-90

[29] Terao C, Matsumura T, Yoshifuji H, Kirino Y, Maejima Y, Nakaoka Y, et al. Takayasu arteritis and ulcerative colitis: high rate of co-occurrence and genetic overlap. Arthritis & Rheumatology (Hoboken, NJ). 2015 May;**67**(8):2226-2232

[30] Scheid R, Teich N. Neurologic manifestations of ulcerative colitis. European Journal of Neurology. 2007 May;**14**(5):483-493

[31] Raj N, Arkebauer M, Waters B, Dickinson B. A case of cerebral vasculitis associated with ulcerative colitis. Case Reports in Rheumatology. 2015;**2015**:598273

[32] Lossos A, River Y, Eliakim A, Steiner I. Neurologic aspects of inflammatory bowel disease. Neurology. 1995 Mar;**45**(3 Pt 1):416-421

[33] Rang EH, Brooke BN, Hermon-Taylor J. Association of ulcerative colitis with multiple sclerosis. Lancet (London, England). 1982 Sep;**2**(8297):555

[34] Marrie RA, Reider N, Cohen J, Stuve O, Sorensen PS, Cutter G, et al. A systematic review of the incidence and prevalence of autoimmune disease in multiple sclerosis. Multiple Sclerosis. 2015 Mar;**21**(3):282-293

[35] Gupta G, Gelfand JM, Lewis JD. Increased risk for demyelinating diseases in patients with inflammatory bowel disease. Gastroenterology. 2005 Sep;**129**(3):819-826

[36] Kosmidou M, Katsanos AH, Katsanos KH, Kyritsis AP, Tsivgoulis G, Christodoulou D, et al. Multiple sclerosis and inflammatory bowel diseases: A systematic review and meta-analysis. Journal of Neurology. 2017 Feb;**264**(2):254-259

[37] Singh S, Kumar N, Loftus EV, Kane SV. Neurologic complications in patients with inflammatory bowel disease: increasing relevance in the era of biologics. Inflammatory Bowel Disease. 2013;**19**(4):864-872

[38] Ramos-Casals M, Roberto-Perez-Alvarez, Diaz-Lagares C, Cuadrado M-J, Khamashta MA, BIOGEAS Study Group. Autoimmune diseases induced by biological agents: A double-edged sword? Autoimmunity Reviews. 2010 Jan;**9**(3):188-93

[39] Mohan N, Edwards ET, Cupps TR, Oliverio PJ, Sandberg G, Crayton H, et al. Demyelination occurring during anti-tumor necrosis factor alpha therapy for inflammatory arthritides. Arthritis and Rheumatism. 2001 Dec;**44**(12):2862-2869

[40] van Oosten BW, Barkhof F, Truyen L, Boringa JB, Bertelsmann FW, von Blomberg BM, et al. Increased MRI activity and immune activation in two multiple sclerosis patients treated with the monoclonal anti-tumor necrosis factor antibody cA2. Neurology. 1996 Dec;**47**(6):1531-1534

[41] Dolapcioglu C, Guleryuzlu Y, Uygur-Bayramicli O, Ahishali E, Dabak R. Asymptomatic brain lesions on cranial magnetic resonance imaging in inflammatory bowel disease. Gut Liver. 2013 Mar;**7**(2):169-174

[42] Hart PE, Gould SR, MacSweeney JE, Clifton A, Schon F. Brain white-matter lesions in inflammatory bowel disease. Lancet (London, England). 1998 May;**351**(9115):1558

[43] Elsehety A, Bertorini TE. Neurologic and neuropsychiatric complications of Crohn's disease. Southern Medical Journal. 1997 Jun;**90**(6):606-610

[44] Masaki T, Muto T, Shinozaki M, Kuroda T. Unusual cerebral complication associated with ulcerative colitis. Journal of Gastroenterology. 1997 Apr;**32**(2):251-254

[45] Fagan C, Phelan D. Severe convulsant hypomagnesaemia and short bowel syndrome. Anaesthesia and Intensive Care. 2001 Jun;**29**(3):281-283

[46] Shorvon S, Andermann F, Guerrini R. The causes of epilepsy. In 2011. pp. 590-1

[47] Benavente L, Morís G. Neurologic disorders associated with inflammatory bowel disease. European Journal of Neurology. 2011;**18**(1):138-143

[48] Gondim FAA, Grannagan TH, Sander HW, Chin RL, Latov N. Peripheral neuropathy in patients with inflammatory bowel disease. Brain. 2005;**128**(4):867-879

[49] Deepak P, Stobaugh DJ, Sherid M, Sifuentes H, Ehrenpreis ED. Neurological events with tumour necrosis factor alpha inhibitors reported to the Food and Drug Administration adverse event reporting system. Alimentary Pharmacology & Therapeutics. 2013 Aug; **38**(4):388-396

[50] Pfeiffer RF. Gastroenterology and neurology. Continuum (Minneap Minn). 2017;**23**(3, Neurology of Systemic Disease):744-61

[51] Morís G. Inflammatory bowel disease: An increased risk factor for neurologic complications. World Journal of Gastroenterology. 2014;**20**(5):1228-1237

[52] Graff LA, Walker JR, Bernstein CN. Depression and anxiety in inflammatory bowel disease: A review of comorbidity and management. Inflammatory Bowel Diseases. 2009 Jul;**15**(7):1105-1118

[53] Nowakowski J, Chrobak AA, Dudek D. Psychiatric illnesses in inflammatory bowel diseases—Psychiatric comorbidity and biological underpinnings. Psychiatria Polska. 2016;**50**(6):1157-1166

[54] Bannaga AS, Selinger CP. Inflammatory bowel disease and anxiety: Links, risks, and challenges faced. Clinical and Experimental Gastroenterology. 2015;**8**:111-117

[55] Panara AJ, Yarur AJ, Rieders B, Proksell S, Deshpande AR, Abreu MT, et al. The incidence and risk factors for developing depression after being diagnosed with inflammatory bowel disease: A cohort study. Alimentary Pharmacology & Therapeutics. 2014 Apr;**39**(8):802-810

[56] Walker JR, Ediger JP, Graff LA, Greenfeld JM, Clara I, Lix L, et al. The Manitoba IBD cohort study: A population-based study of the prevalence of lifetime and 12-month anxiety and mood disorders. The American Journal of Gastroenterology. 2008 Aug;**103**(8): 1989-1997

[57] Eaton WW, Pedersen MG, Nielsen PR, Mortensen PB. Autoimmune diseases, bipolar disorder, and non-affective psychosis. Bipolar Disorders. 2010 Sep;**12**(6):638-646

[58] Bonaz BL, Bernstein CN. Brain-gut interactions in inflammatory bowel disease. Gastroenterology. 2013 Jan;**144**(1):36-49

[59] Benarroch EE. The central autonomic network: Functional organization, dysfunction, and perspective. Mayo Clinic Proceedings. 1993 Oct;**68**(10):988-1001

[60] Ghia J-E, Blennerhassett P, Deng Y, Verdu EF, Khan WI, Collins SM. Reactivation of inflammatory bowel disease in a mouse model of depression. Gastroenterology. 2009 Jun;**136**(7):2280-8.e1-4

[61] Martin-Subero M, Anderson G, Kanchanatawan B, Berk M, Maes M. Comorbidity between depression and inflammatory bowel disease explained by immune-inflammatory, oxidative, and nitrosative stress; tryptophan catabolite; and gut-brain pathways. CNS Spectrums. 2016 Apr;**21**(2):184-198

Section 4

Therapy of Inflammatory Bowel Disease

Chapter 4

Nutritional Therapy for Inflammatory Bowel Disease

Rok Orel, Evgen Benedik, Janez Eržen,
Anija Orel and Darja Urlep

Additional information is available at the end of the chapter

http://dx.doi.org/10.5772/intechopen.73259

Abstract

The components of a diet influence intestinal microbiota, epithelial barrier function, immune system, and many other factors that play important role in both development and treatment of inflammation in gastrointestinal tract. We briefly review potential role of specific dietary compounds as a risk or protective factor, but we predominantly concentrate on nutritional status and nutritional intervention in patients with inflammatory bowel disease. Besides exclusive enteral nutrition as a potential first-line treatment in active Crohn's disease, other nutritional therapeutic modalities such as partial enteral nutrition, parenteral nutrition, diets based on carbohydrate modifications, anti-inflammatory diet, and the use of specific dietary compounds with anti-inflammatory properties, known as pharmaconutrition, are presented.

Keywords: inflammatory bowel disease, Crohn's disease, ulcerative colitis, nutrition, nutritional therapy

1. Introduction

The exact etiology and pathophysiologic mechanisms of inflammatory bowel diseases (IBD) are not completely explained, but the complex interplay among genetic background, environmental factors, intestinal microbiota, and immune system seems to be implemented. The incidence and prevalence of both types of IBD, Crohn's disease (CD) and ulcerative colitis (UC), has dramatically increased in western countries and in developed Asian countries in the last 50 years [1]. In addition, several epidemiologic studies revealed that the incidence of IBD in descendants of immigrants from the parts of the world with low incidence to the countries with high incidence resembles the one of the native population and not of the county of their origin [2, 3]; these points to the crucial role of environmental factors/changes in IBD epidemics. The potential influences of specific factors such as changes in hygiene/sanitation, decreased exposure to infectious agents, smoking, water and air pollution, psychological stress, and an increased use of certain drugs have all been proposed and are reviewed elsewhere [4, 5]. An increasing body of evidence is linking IBD with diet.

Dietary constituents and their proportions can affect human physiology directly. However, intestinal microbiota, recently recognized as an essential component of metabolism, immune and neuroendocrine regulation, is also importantly influenced by diet. For example, intestinal microbiota of African children, whose diet is based on fiber-rich, plant-derived diet, was found to be vastly different to microbiota of their European peers, who consume diet rich in sugar, diary, fat, and protein [6]. Animal studies revealed that change from low-fat, high-fiber diet to "Western style" diet rich in fat and sugar resulted in substantial shift in microbiota within a single day [7]. Changes in composition and function of intestinal microbiota because of specific dietary patterns may lead to a state not favorable for host organism, defined as dysbiosis. Numerous studies have shown that gut microbiota of IBD patients substantially differs from the one of healthy individuals and that these changes may play a crucial role in the development and activity of the disease [8]. Enteric microbiota plays an essential role in metabolizing nutrients, especially those not completely digestible by human digestive enzymes, such as fiber, resulting in production of diversity of biologically active components, such as short chain fatty acids (SCFAs) and intestinal gases. A study from Japan showed that people living in rural areas consuming traditional Japanese food have more abundant Bifidobacteria, which are recognized as an important producer of SCFAs, than urban population eating western-type diet [9]. Western-type diets, rich in saturated fat and protein and poor in plant fiber, result in depletion of Firmicutes, which are involved in metabolism of plant polysaccharides, and decrease in SCFA production [10]. On the other hand, this kind of diet promotes growth of proteolytic bacteria, such as Bilophila wadsworthia and other bile tolerant microbes, which use proteins and bile acids as a source of organic sulfur and produce hydrogen sulfide (H2S). H2S can be genotoxic, modulate expression in cell cycle progression, trigger inflammatory response, and impair DNA repair [8].

Direct effects of relative abundancy/deficiency of specific nutrients and changes in composition and functioning of intestinal microbiota can lead to impairment of intestinal barrier function, including decreased resistance to invasion of pathobionts, dysfunction of innate, and adaptive immune system that finally results in chronic inflammation and tissue damage characteristic for IBD.

In this chapter, we try to review current knowledge about the effects of specific food components on IBD concentrating on clinical evidence about efficacy of different dietary interventions in IBD patients.

2. Role of specific food constituents

Most of our knowledge about the influence of specific food ingredients on intestinal function, development of inflammation, and IBD in particular originates either from animal model experiments or from epidemiological studies.

2.1. Fats

There is a growing evidence that some types of fat act pro-inflammatory, while the others protect against development of intestinal inflammation. Several big epidemiologic studies, such as European Investigation into Cancer and Nutrition Study (EPIC) and the Nurses' Health Study have pointed to an increased risk of IBD among people who consume greater amounts of meat and fats, particularly polyunsaturated fatty acids and omega-6 fatty acids [11–13]. The EPIC study revealed an association between greater consumption of an omega-6 polyunsaturated fatty acid (PUFA), linoleic acid, present in high concentrations in red meat, cooking oils, and margarine and higher incidence of UC. In contrast, people who consumed higher levels of omega-3 PUFA docosahexaenoic acid (DHA) were less likely to develop UC [11–13]. Similarly, consumption of large quantities of nuts and fish, which are rich in omega-3 PUFA such as DHA, eicosapentaenoic acid (EPA), and docosapentaenoic acid (DPA), was shown to lower the risk for CD [14]. Omega-3 fatty acids were shown to have an anti-inflammatory, antithrombotic, antiarrhythmic, and hypolipemic effect [15]. There was also a significantly reduced risk for CD when ratio of long-chain omega-3/arachidonic acid was high in the consumed food [14].

In conclusion, it seems that diet rich in animal fats and particularly omega-6 PUFA promotes dysbiosis and intestinal inflammation that may lead to development of IBD in genetically susceptible hosts. On the other hand, omega-3 PUFA seems to play a protective role and may even promote anti-inflammatory mechanisms.

2.2. Proteins

As already mentioned, several epidemiologic studies revealed an association between consumption of large quantities of meat and increased risk for IBD [11–13]. It is not clear whether this association was only due to increased intake of fats or also of proteins, as the results of the studies regarding the role of proteins in IBD were conflicting [13]. In one study, high intake of proteins found in meat but not in dairy products was found to be positively associated with IBD [16].

Among the specific proteins and peptides, the effects of gluten-derived proteins were particularly attentive. In animal model, gluten-fortified experimental diet induced chronic ileitis [17]. They found reduced occludin expression levels, and these findings suggest a negative role of gluten on intestinal barrier integrity. Experiments on intestinal epithelial cell lines showed that gliadin induces an increase in intestinal permeability due to zonulin release by binding to the chemokine receptor CXCR3 [18]. Zonulin is the physiologic modulator of tight junctions that regulate intestinal permeability through the epithelial paracellular pathway. Its upregulation in genetically susceptible individuals may lead to different immune-mediated diseases [19]. It was observed that intestinal permeability increased after gliadin exposure not only in patients with celiac disease or nonceliac gluten sensitivity but, although to a lesser extent, also in healthy subjects [20].

2.3. Carbohydrates

Many epidemiological studies pointed out that excessive consumption of simple carbohydrates, refined sugars, sweet carbonized drinks, or even artificial sweeteners might represent a risk factor for the development of IBD; however, as many others failed to prove this association [21]. Individual studies even showed that low complex carbohydrates and low refined sugar intake significantly improved laboratory inflammatory markers and fecal calprotectin in patients with IDB [22].

On the other hand, consummation of vegetables and fruits rich in both soluble and insoluble fiber has been shown to be negatively associated with IBD [14, 23, 24]. Animal studies confirmed that plant polysaccharides and poorly digestible fibrous plant components have reduced features of experimental colitis [25]. Fermentable fiber is fermented by saccharolytic gut microbiota, resulting in increased production of SCFAs. SCFAs, especially butyrate, are utilized not only as fuel sources for colonocyte that results in enhancement of the intestinal barrier, but also possess anti-inflammatory effect, mainly through inhibition of the production and release of inflammatory mediators [26, 27]. In addition, some vegetables like broccoli and cabbage are thought to activate the aryl hydrocarbon receptor (AhR), which is highly expressed by intestinal intraepithelial lymphocytes and is involved in immune regulation and defense against attacks of luminal microorganisms [28]. Overall, refined and processed carbohydrates and intake of sweetened beverages are thought to be risk factors for developing IBD, while complex carbohydrates like vegetables, fruit, and fiber showed to be protective.

2.4. Food additives

It has been hypothesized that emulsifiers, detergent-like molecules that are a ubiquitous component of processed foods, can disrupt intestinal mucus layer, increase intestinal permeability, and enable bacterial translocation across epithelia [29]. In mice, relatively low concentrations of two commonly used emulsifiers, carboxymethylcellulose and polysorbate-80, induced low-grade inflammation in wild-type hosts and promoted robust colitis in mice predisposed to IBD [30].

Maltodextrin, a polysaccharide derived from starch hydrolysis, was found to promote adherent-invasive E coli (AIEC) biofilms and increase adhesion of AIEC strains to intestinal epithelial cells and macrophages [31]. Strains of AIEC have been isolated from the ileum and the colon of CD patients [32, 33].

Therefore, consumption of maltodextrin and emulsifiers may possibly support growth of intestinal pathobionts, such as AIEC and their translocation across epithelial barrier, where they could survive in macrophages and lead to chronic inflammation.

3. Nutritional status of IBD patients

According to available data, malnutrition affects 65–75% of patients with CD and 18–62% of patients with UC [34, 35]. In pediatric IBD patients, malnutrition frequently results not only in weight loss but also in growth retardation [36, 37].

Main reason for malnutrition in IBD patients is insufficient food intake due to the loss of appetite and avoidance of certain foods presumably worsening the symptoms, resulting in prolonged restrictive diets [38, 39]. Intestinal inflammation and inflammatory cytokines released from immune cells can damage epithelial integrity and impair absorption of nutrients. In addition, bacterial overgrowth and increased intestinal mobility may contribute to malabsorption [40, 41]. Fat and fat-soluble vitamin absorption may be especially impaired in CD patients when terminal ileum is seriously affected due to the biliary salt malabsorption [42]. Some of the medications used for IBD treatment, such as glucocorticoids, sulfasalazine, and immune system suppressants, could have a negative impact on micronutrient absorption and utilization [34, 42]. It should be noted that IBD patients with active inflammation have increased metabolic rate, which leads to increased energy expenditure [36, 37, 43].

An important aspect of malnutrition in IBD patients is alteration of body composition. Fat mass (FM) consists of adipose tissues (both visceral and subcutaneous) while fat-free mass (FFM) consists of water, proteins, minerals, and other components [35]. Clinical studies revealed an important reduction of both FM and FFM in active phase of IBD. However, it was also reported that FM was frequently recovered during remission phase, while FFM remained depleted [35].

Malnutrition, immobility, low protein synthesis, and increased proteolysis due to inflammation are the main mechanisms leading to sarcopenia, a progressive and generalized loss of skeletal muscle mass and strength with risk of poor quality of life and physical disability [44]. Sarcopenia has various negative health consequences such as pathological fractures due to bone demineralization, cardiovascular disease, and higher probability of hospitalization [44].

Several studies reported that despite aforementioned causes leading to malnutrition in IBD, one-third of the patients are obese, the proportion is similar in CD and UC patients [45, 46]. Obese IBD patients do not have worst long-term clinical outcome than normal weight patients [47]. However, simultaneous presence of sarcopenia and obesity, so-called sarcopenic obesity, is related to a fast functional decline of patient's status, with a high risk of morbidity, disability, and mortality [44].

Micronutrient and vitamin deficiencies are common in IBD patients. Preventions of those deficiencies are mandatory for avoidance of possible clinical complications. The most common micronutrient deficiencies described in IBD patients are known for iron, calcium, selenium, zinc, magnesium, and vitamins, in particular B12, folic acid, A, D, and K [34, 42].

One of the important features of IBD is anemia. Its prevalence in pediatric patients is up to 70% and in adult patients up to 50% [48]. The most frequent cause of anemia in IBD patients is iron deficiency (prevalence estimated in 36–90% of CD and UC patients), following vitamin B12 (prevalence estimated in 22% of CD and 3% of UC patients) [34, 49], and folic acid (vitamin B9) deficiencies (prevalence estimated in 29% of CD and 9% of UC patients) [50]. These deficiencies are the consequence of bleeding from mucosal lesions, inadequate dietary intake, impaired absorption and utilization, surgery (ileal resection greater than 60 cm will develop B12 deficiency), systemic inflammation, and medications [37, 50, 51].

Calcium and Vitamin D deficiency are often in IBD patients, especially in those with duodenal and jejunal disease, when their absorption is disturbed [34, 42]. Their prevalence is 70% in CD and 40% in UC patients. Besides its influence on bone metabolism, vitamin D have important role in preserving mucosal integrity and mucosal healing capacity. In case of its deficiency, the risk for mucosal damage and for IBD is higher [34, 42]. It was shown that high levels of active vitamin D not only reduce the risk of developing CD, but also the risk of developing UC [52, 53].

Vitamin A deficiency in IBD patients is high up to 90%. Vitamin A deficiency results in impaired wound healing, night blindness, and xerophthalmia [34, 42].

Vitamin K deficiency in IBD patients is also reported, but the prevalence is unknown. Most important source of vitamin K is intestinal production by gut microbiota. Dysbiosis, use of antibiotics, and malabsorption may contribute to this deficiency [34, 42].

Inadequate dietary intake and chronic loss because of diarrhea are the main reasons for selenium, zinc, and magnesium deficiencies in IBD patients for which the exact prevalence is not known. Symptoms associated with deficiencies include bone health impairment, cartilage degeneration, fatigue, and poor wound healing [34, 42].

4. Nutritional intervention

EEN has been evaluated in a number of clinical studies including randomized controlled trials (RCTs) that compared EEN to CS in adult and pediatric populations of patients with active CD. To date, eight meta-analyses have been published on the efficacy of EEN versus CS. Among these meta-analyses, three of them were performed exclusively on the pediatric population while others included adult patients as well. While meta-analyses of adult studies have suggested better efficacy of CS, pediatric studies have shown that EEN is at least as effective as CS in inducing remission and is superior to CS in improving nutritional status and growth recovery without adverse side effects [54].

The main goals of nutritional intervention in IBD patients are treatment and prevention of malnutrition, treatment of active inflammation and maintaining remission in Crohn's disease, and symptomatic treatment in specific situations [55].

Regular evaluation of nutritional status, early detection of specific deficits and specific risk factors are crucial for adequate nutritional treatment. Anthropometric measurements and basic laboratory tests, such as hemoglobin concentration and markers of inflammation, should be checked regularly at every visit, while the frequency of albumin, ferritin, vitamin, and trace element concentration checkout depends on the activity of the disease, but should be done at least once a year when the disease is quiescent [55]. Periodical evaluation of detailed body composition and bone mineral density is recommended. Bioimpedance (BIA) and dual-energy X-ray absorptiometry (DEXA) are considered as the gold standard for measuring body composition [56]. A dietary history and, sometimes, prospective dietary record are necessary to get a good estimate of food intake. We should be aware that many patients develop special dietary habits due to their belief that consumption of specific foods (e.g., dairy, meat, fruit, and vegetables) results in symptoms or even worsen the disease course, which may additionally contribute to the development of nutritional deficiencies [57].

With the exception of the ECCO/ESPGHAN recommendations to use exclusive enteral nutrition as a first-line therapeutic approach in children with active CD [58], the strict guidelines for nutritional intervention in IBD does not exist. However, many different dietary approaches have been developed and studied, with intention to alleviate patients' symptoms or even treat the disease.

4.1. Exclusive and partial enteral nutrition

Exclusive enteral nutrition (EEN) means that 100% of a person's nutritional requirements is provided by a liquid nutritional formula either orally or via a feeding tube. Numerous studies have shown that the treatment of active CD with exclusive enteral nutrition (EEN), especially in children, is as effective as corticosteroids in inducing remission. EEN, used as monotherapy, can induce remission in up to 80% of patients with active CD [59, 60]. It is well established that treatment with EEN is capable of achieving mucosal healing. On the contrary, corticosteroids have poor ability to induce mucosal healing [61]. In comparison to therapy with drugs, EEN has no adverse effects and, even more importantly, improves growth, and reverses malnutrition [58]. Therefore, according to the ECCO/ESPGHAN guidelines for treatment of pediatric CD patients, EEN is recommended as a first-line treatment in children and adolescents with active CD [58]. Meta-analysis of the results of the studies using ENN for the therapy of active CD in adult CD patients indicated that it was less effective than steroids in inducing remission; however, this conclusion was based on intention-to-treat analysis [62]. However, when only the results of the patients who completed the course of EEN were analyzed, the remission rates were comparable to those achieved by steroids [63].

EEN is usually provided for 6–8 week, and then a normal diet is gradually reintroduced. Enteral formulas are differentiated by the structure of their protein content. Elemental diets contain no intact protein, but only amino acids. Semielemental diets are based on peptides of varying lengths. Polymeric formulas contain whole proteins and are therefore more palatable in comparison with elemental diets [64]. Protocols of EEN may be different regarding the composition of the enteral formula and route of administration. Elemental diets often require a feeding tube to administer due to their poor palatability. In addition, polymeric formulas are reported to cost less. Various studies and a large meta-analysis later demonstrated that polymeric formulas were as effective as elemental formulas [65].

Although EEN has been shown to be efficacious, its mechanism of action remains unknown. Possible mechanisms include a change in gut microbiota, bowel rest, dietary antigen elimination, improvement in the nutritional status, and potential anti-inflammatory properties of specific ingredients of enteral formulas. Currently, the modification of gut microbiota seems to be the most probable proposed mechanism for ENN efficacy. The next very important mechanism may be associated with exclusion of potentially harmful food ingredients [60].

One of the proposed challenges influencing acceptance of EEN is the restriction of other oral food intake, which may seriously limit compliance with the EEN protocol [66]. Therefore, studies on partial enteral nutrition (PEN), which allows patients with active CD to consume a part of their daily caloric needs from a normal diet, have been conducted.

The results reported from the first study on the efficacy of PEN did not indicate that PEN providing 50% of caloric needs by formula was effective for induction of remission in pediatric CD [67]. However, the results of some recently published studies are more promising. Israeli authors combined PEN with Crohn's Disease Exclusion Diet (CDED) [68]. CDED is a structured diet, which excludes animal fats, milk and dairy, gluten, and all processed and canned foods, which contain additives, especially emulsifiers and maltodextrin. The authors hypothesize that the major mechanism leading to response to EEN used in children with active CD is exclusion of specific dietary factors, which may have a negative impact on mucous layer, intestinal permeability, and colonization with adherent-invasive E coli (AIEC). The study protocol allowed patients to consume up to 50% daily calories from CDED. Response and remission were obtained in 78.7 and 70.2% patients, respectively. Different approaches using PEN was developed at the Children's Hospital of Philadelphia [69]. The patients receive 80–90% of their energy input from EN, but they were allowed to consume remaining calories from a normal diet. Retrospective analysis revealed remission rate of 65% and response rate of 87%, which is comparable with the remission rates from the studies using EEN. Further studies are needed to elucidate the efficacy of this treatment approach.

One of the problems of CD therapy with EEN is that disease relapses relatively frequently soon after stopping EN when the patients are not receiving maintenance therapy. Several studies using PEP as a maintenance therapy either alone or in combination with drugs were performed in both pediatric and adult patients with CD. The results of the majority of these studies, as well as their systematic reviews [70–72], showed that the relapse rate during observational period was significantly lower in patients using PEP compared with those consuming regular unrestricted diet and that efficacy of maintenance therapy with PEP might be comparable to standard therapy with drugs. In addition, nutritional status as well as linear growth of children with CD was found to be better in those using PEP during remission in comparison with patients on regular diet [73].

4.2. Total parenteral nutrition

In the 1980s, total parenteral nutrition (TPN) was used to treat patients with moderate to severe CD. The aim of TPN as primary therapy for IBD was to achieve bowel rest, to correct nutritional deficits, and to remove antigenic mucosal stimuli [74, 75]. In the 1990s, treatment with exclusive enteral nutrition (EEN) was shown to have similar or even better results in terms of remission rate in active CD disease. When TPN and ENN are compared, TPN is associated with higher costs and significant risk of serious adverse events including sepsis. Therefore, TPN should be restricted to patients who cannot be adequately fed by enteral route, mainly those with gut failure and short-bowel syndrome [76].

According to recent ESPEN guidelines on clinical nutrition in IBD, TPN is indicated only when EN has failed or it is impossible to be administered [77].

4.3. Diets based on carbohydrate modifications

Low-fiber or even so-called low-residue diets are frequently recommended during acute exacerbations of IBD [78]. While a low-fiber diet excludes only insoluble fiber, a low-residue diet requires exclusion of not only all vegetables, fruits, whole grains, legumes, but also dairy products and fibrous meat [79]. A basic idea behind these diets is that they reduce the volume and frequency of stools as well as the risk of intestinal obstruction. Although these diets are usually prescribed for a short-term use, many patients continue with them for a long period of time. Objective studies failed to find any difference in severity of symptoms, number of complications, and needs for hospitalization or surgery between patients using such diets and those consuming unrestricted diet [80]. As already mentioned, indigestible carbohydrates, especially the fermentable ones may play an important protective role in IBD, as they represent the main substrate for production of SCFAs by intestinal bacteria. The only patients that may benefit from fiber restriction are those with strictures and obstructive symptoms.

Significant proportion of IBD patients also suffers from functional irritable bowel syndrome-like symptoms even in remission independently of actual level of the inflammation [81]. Low fermentable oligosaccharide, disaccharide, monosaccharide, and polyol (FODMAP) diet results in symptom relief in many of such patients [82]. However, low-FODMAP diet is very restrictive, so it should be carefully planned by professional dietetics to prevent development of specific nutritional deficiencies. In addition, the influence of low-FODMAP diet on the microbiome, metabolism, and inflammation in patients with IBD is still unclear.

On the other side, several studies using fiber-rich supplements such as wheat or oat bran [83, 84], psyllium [85, 86], and germinated barley foodstuff [87, 88] revealed their efficacy in symptomatic improvement and in decreasing disease activity indices either in CD or UC patients. Moreover, reduced concentrations of inflammatory cytokines, such as TNF-α, IL-6, and IL-8, pointed to the possible anti-inflammatory effect of dietary fiber, probably through their influence on microbiota and SCFA production [89].

Another diet, based mainly not only on restriction of specific carbohydrates but also on some other foods, called the specific carbohydrate diet (SCD) was developed in the 1920s [90]. Since then, this diet has been used in a variety of different conditions, including IBD, irritable bowel syndrome, celiac disease, and autism [91]. The SCD restricts all carbohydrates except monosaccharides: glucose, fructose, and galactose. This diet is based on a hypothesis that complex carbohydrates may induce intestinal dysbiosis resulting in the development of inflammation [92]. While fresh or cooked fruits, vegetables, and legumes are in general acceptable, all grains as well as potatoes should be omitted. In more restrictive versions of SCD, even milk and dairy products, refined sugar and artificial sweeteners, corn, and maple syrup are prohibited. In addition, all-otherwise permitted food should not be processed (canned, smoked, etc.) and should not contain potentially harmful additives [91]. Several relatively small studies found out that SCD alone without taking medications may lead to clinical improvement, reflected by symptom disappearance and significant reduction of laboratory markers of inflammation, in some patient with active CD [91, 93]. However, recently published study using endoscopic evaluation before and after the treatment with SCD revealed that despite some clinical effect, complete mucosal healing was never achieved [94].

4.4. IBD-anti-inflammatory diet

Recently, an investigator group from USA developed the IBD-anti-inflammatory diet (IBD-AID) to be offered to IBD patients who are refractory to pharmacological therapy, or for whom the treatment is not as effective as desired [95]. The IBD-AID has five basic components. The first is the restriction of certain carbohydrates, including lactose, and refined or processed complex carbohydrates. The second is the use of pre- and probiotics and foods rich in the components that help to restore the balance of the intestinal microbiota (e.g., soluble fiber, leeks, onions, and fermented foods). The third is distinctive use of saturated, trans-, mono-, and polyunsaturated fats. The fourth principle is to review the overall dietary pattern, detect missing nutrients, and identify specific food intolerances. The last component is a modification of food textures to improve absorption of nutrients and to minimize the adverse effect of intact fiber. In practice, the IBD-AID consists of lean meats, poultry, fish, omega-3 eggs, particular sources of carbohydrates, select fruits and vegetables, nuts, and legume flours, but restricts the consumption of wheat, rye, and barley products as well as milk and dairy products other than yogurt, kefir, and limited aged cheeses. A retrospective review of their case series including both patients with CD and UC revealed that approximately one-third of the patients chose not to attempt this diet, while the vast majority of those who followed the diet for 4 weeks or more reported symptom reduction and were able to discontinue at least one of their prior IBD medications [95]. However, randomized clinical trials are needed to properly elucidate the efficacy of this treatment regimen.

4.5. Pharmaconutrition

Several studies have shown that specific nutrients when supplemented in quantities exceeding their nutritional role may affect the immune system, metabolism, and gastrointestinal structure and function. Such examples are some amino acids like glutamine, arginine and tryptophan [96], omega-3 PUFA [97], vitamin D [98], and curcumin [99].

Glutamine and arginine are thought to be immunomodulatory and could be involved in mediating responses to metabolic stress. Studies on animal models revealed that they improved biochemical and clinical parameters of chemical-induced colitis [100]. Histamine, a biogenic amine derived from the amino acid histidine, reduced symptoms of experimental immune-mediated colitis [101]. Similarly, threonine reduced features of colitis and enhanced intestinal mucus production, which in turn leads to better barrier function [102, 103]. Tryptophan, another essential amino acid, also possesses strong anti-inflammatory effect both by direct action on intestinal and immune system cells and indirectly serves as a precursor for serotonin and melatonin [103]. A detailed review on the effects of specific amino acids on intestinal inflammation can be found elsewhere [96]. Although these amino acids may have some positive effect in IBD patients, their efficacy has not been adequately studied yet.

Omega-3 PUFA negatively affects intestinal inflammation through several mechanisms. [97]. They can act as a substrate for anti-inflammatory eicosanoid production, as well as a substrate for the synthesis of resolvins, maresins, and protectins, engaged in resolution of inflammatory process. On the other hand, they reduce production of pro-inflammatory cytokines such as TNF-α, decrease expression of adhesion molecules and possess antioxidative and chemoprotective properties. The results of clinical trials using omega-3 PUFA in patients with either CD or UC were inconsistent. Cochrane review, considering the use of omega-3 PUFA for maintenance treatment published in 2011, revealed a small but significant benefit in CD, but not in UC patients [104].

Besides its role in calcium metabolism and bone mineralization, vitamin D is regarded as an important anti-inflammatory agent. It regulates immune cells trafficking and differentiation, intestinal permeability, and antimicrobial peptide synthesis [98]. Several studies revealed an inverse association between serum concentration of 25-hydroxy-vitamin D and mucosal inflammation in IBD patients [105, 106]. Therefore, supplementation in IBD patients with low serum level of vitamin D seems mandatory. In a randomized controlled trial, a maintenance dose of 1200 IU/day, regardless of vitamin D status at entry, reduced a relapse rate in patients with CD [107].

Curcumin is the active compound found in turmeric. It possesses anti-inflammatory, anti-oxidant, anticancer, and neuroprotective properties [99]. Several studies and systematic reviews reveal that supplementation with curcumin when provided simultaneously with medications is both effective and a safe option for maintenance treatment of UC [108, 109].

5. Conclusion

Nutritional intervention is an important part of the treatment in IBD patients. Goals of nutritional intervention exceed provision of energy, macronutrients, and micronutrients to ensure adequate nutritional status of the patients. Recognition of the ability of specific food ingredients to interfere with the disease mechanisms has led to the development of several therapeutic approaches based on a diet modification. However, only the effectiveness of exclusive enteral nutrition in active CD has been proven enough to find place in different international therapeutic guidelines. As this kind of diet is difficult to keep for a prolonged period of time, other potential options such as partial enteral nutrition and restriction or even exclusion of potentially harmful foods with simultaneous increased intake of food ingredients that potentially interfere with different pathologic mechanisms seem extremely promising. However, we need to confirm the efficacy and safety of these novel dietary approaches more firmly before recommending their routine use in an everyday clinical practice.

Conflict of interest

Authors have no conflict of interest.

Author details

Rok Orel[1]*, Evgen Benedik[1], Janez Eržen[1], Anija Orel[2] and Darja Urlep[1]

*Address all correspondence to: rok.orel@kclj.si

1 University Children's Hospital, University Medical Centre Ljubljana, Ljubljana, Slovenia

2 Clinical Nutrition Unit, Institute of Oncology Ljubljana, Ljubljana, Slovenia

References

[1] Bernstein CN. Review article: Changes in the epidemiology of inflammatory bowel disease—Clues for aetiology. Alimentary Pharmacology & Therapeutics. 2017;**46**:911-919. DOI: 10.1111/apt.14338

[2] Walker DG, Williams HRT, Kane SP, Mawdsley JE, Arnold J, McNeil I, et al. Differences in inflammatory bowel disease phenotype between south Asians and northern Europeans living in north West London, UK. The American Journal of Gastroenterology. 2011;**106**:1281-1289. DOI: 10.1038/ajg.2011.85

[3] Li X, Sundquist J, Hemminki K, Sundquist K. Risk of inflammatory bowel disease in first- and second-generation immigrants in Sweden: A nationwide follow-up study. Inflammatory Bowel Diseases. 2011;**17**:1784-1791. DOI: 10.1002/ibd.21535

[4] Dutta AK, Chacko A. Inflammatory Bowel Disease: Global view influence of environmental factors on the onset and course of inflammatory bowel disease. World Journal of Gastroenterology. 2016;**22**:1088-1100. DOI: 10.3748/wjg.v22.i3.1088

[5] Abegunde AT, Muhammad BH, Bhatti O, Ali T. Environmental risk factors for inflammatory bowel diseases: Evidence based literature review. World Journal of Gastroenterology. 2016;**22**:6296-6317. DOI: 10.3748/wjg.v22.i27.6296

[6] De Filippo C, Cavalieri D, Di Paola M, Ramazzotti M, Poullet JB, Massart S, et al. Impact of diet in shaping gut microbiota revealed by a comparative study in children from Europe and rural Africa. Proceedings of the National Academy of Sciences. 2010;**107**:14691-14696. DOI: 10.1073/pnas.1005963107

[7] Turnbaugh PJ, Ridaura VK, Faith JJ, Rey FE, Knight R, Gordon JI. The effect of diet on the human gut Microbiom: A metagenomic analysis in humanized Gnotobiotic mice. Science Translational Medicine. 2009;**1**:1-19. DOI: 10.1126/scitranslmed.3000322.The

[8] Leone, VA Cham, CM Chang E. Diet, gut microbes, and genetics in immune function: Can we leverage our current knowledge to achieve better outcomes in inflammatory bowel diseases? Current Opinion in Immunology. 2014:16-23. DOI:10.1016/j.jnutbio.2013.01.006. Nutritional

[9] Benno Y, Suzuki K, Suzuki K, Narisawa K, Bruce WR, Mitsuoka T. Comparison of the fecal microflora in rural Japanese and urban Canadians. Microbiology and Immunology. 1986;**30**:521-532. DOI: 10.1111/j.1348-0421.1986.tb02978.x

[10] David LA, Maurice CF, Carmody RN, Gootenberg DB, Button JE, Wolfe BE, et al. Diet rapidly and reproducibly alters the human gut microbiome. Nature. 2014;**505**:559-563. DOI: 10.1038/nature12820.Diet

[11] Tjonneland A, Overvad K, Bergmann M, Nagel G, Linseisen J, Hallmans G, et al. Linoleic acid, a dietary n-6 polyunsaturated fatty acid, and the aetiology of ulcerative colitis: A nested case-control study within a European prospective cohort study. Gut. 2009;**58**:1606-1611. DOI: 10.1136/gut.2008.169078

[12] Ananthakrishnan AN, Khalili H, Konijeti GG, Higuchi LM, de Silva P, Fuchs CS, et al. Long-term intake of dietary fat and risk of ulcerative colitis and Crohn's disease. Gut. 2014;**63**:776-784. DOI:10.1136/gutjnl-2013-305304

[13] Hou JK, Abraham B, El-Serag H. Dietary intake and risk of developing inflammatory bowel disease: A systematic review of the literature. The American Journal of Gastroenterology. 2011;**106**:563-573. DOI: 10.1038/ajg.2011.44

[14] Amre DK, D'Souza S, Morgan K, Seidman G, Lambrette P, Grimard G, et al. Imbalances in dietary consumption of fatty acids, vegetables, and fruits are associated with risk for Crohn's disease in children. The American Journal of Gastroenterology. 2007;**102**:2016-2025. DOI: 10.1111/j.1572-0241.2007.01411.x

[15] Akabas SR, Deckelbaum RJ. Summary of a workshop on n-3 fatty acids: Current status of recommendations and future directions. The American Journal of Clinical Nutrition. 2006;**83**:1536S-1538S

[16] Jantchou P, Morois S, Clavel-Chapelon F, Boutron-Ruault M-C, Carbonnel F. Animal protein intake and risk of inflammatory bowel disease: The E3N prospective study. The American Journal of Gastroenterology. 2010;**105**:2195-2201. DOI: 10.1038/ajg.2010.192

[17] Wagner SJ, Schmidt A, Effenberger MJP, Gruber L, Danier J, Haller D. Semisynthetic diet ameliorates Crohn's disease-like ileitis in TNFDeltaARE/WT mice through antigen-independent mechanisms of gluten. Inflammatory Bowel Diseases. 2013;**19**:1285-1294. DOI: 10.1097/MIB.0b013e318281f573

[18] Lammers KM. Lu R, Brownley J, Lu B, Gerard C, Rallabhandi P, et al. gliadin induces an increase in intestinal permeability and zonulin release by binding to the chemokine receptor CXCR3. Gastroenterology. 2009;**135**:194-204. DOI: 10.1053/j.gastro.2008.03.023. Gliadin

[19] Fasano A. Zonulin, regulation of tight junctions, and autoimmune diseases. Annals of the New York Academy of Sciences. 2012;**1258**:25-33. DOI: 10.1111/j.1749-6632.2012.06538.x

[20] Hollon J, Puppa EL, Greenwald B, Goldberg E, Guerrerio A, Fasano A. Effect of gliadin on permeability of intestinal biopsy explants from celiac disease patients and patients with non-celiac gluten sensitivity. Nutrients. 2015;**7**:1565-1576. DOI: 10.3390/nu7031565

[21] Spooren CEGM, Pierik MJ, Zeegers MP, Feskens EJM, Masclee AAM, Jonkers DMAE. Review article: The association of diet with onset and relapse in patients with inflammatory bowel disease. Alimentary Pharmacology & Therapeutics. 2013;**38**:1172-1187. DOI: 10.1111/apt.12501

[22] Lee D, Baldassano RN, Otley AR, Albenberg L, Griffiths AM, Compher C, et al. Comparative effectiveness of nutritional and biological therapy in north American children with active Crohn's disease. Inflammatory Bowel Diseases. 2015;**21**:1786-1793. DOI: 10.1097/MIB.0000000000000426

[23] Ananthakrishnan AN, Khalili H, Konijeti GG, Higuchi LM, de Silva P, Korzenik JR, et al. A prospective study of long-term intake of dietary fiber and risk of Crohn's disease and ulcerative colitis. Gastroenterology. 2013;**145**:970-977. DOI:10.1053/j.gastro.2013.07.050

[24] D'Souza S, Levy E, Mack D, Israel D, Lambrette P, Ghadirian P, et al. Dietary patterns and risk for Crohn's disease in children. Inflammatory Bowel Diseases. 2008;**14**:367-373. DOI: 10.1002/ibd.20333

[25] Nanau RM, Neuman MG. Nutritional and probiotic supplementation in colitis models. Digestive Diseases and Sciences. 2012;**57**:2786-2810. DOI: 10.1007/s10620-012-2284-3

[26] Galvez J, Rodriguez-Cabezas ME, Zarzuelo A. Effects of dietary fiber on inflammatory bowel disease. Molecular Nutrition & Food Research. 2005;**49**:601-608. DOI: 10.1002/mnfr.200500013

[27] Andoh A, Tsujikawa T, Fujiyama Y. Role of dietary fiber and short-chain fatty acids in the colon. Current Pharmaceutical Design. 2003;**9**:347-358

[28] Monteleone I, Pallone F, Monteleone G. Aryl hydrocarbon receptor and colitis. Seminars in Immunopathology. 2013;**35**:671-675. DOI: 10.1007/s00281-013-0396-2

[29] Sarbagili-Shabat C, Sigall-Boneh R, Levine A. Nutritional therapy in inflammatory bowel disease. Current Opinion in Gastroenterology. 2015;**31**:303-308. DOI: 10.1097/MOG.0000000000000178

[30] Chassaing B, Koren O, Goodrich JK, Poole AC, Srinivasan S, Ley RE, et al. Dietary emulsifiers impact the mouse gut microbiota promoting colitis and metabolic syndrome. Nature. 2015;**519**:92-96

[31] Nickerson KP, McDonald C. Crohn's disease-associated adherent-invasive Escherichia Coli adhesion is enhanced by exposure to the ubiquitous dietary polysaccharide maltodextrin. PLoS One. 2012;**7**:e52132

[32] Rahman K, Sasaki M, Nusrat A, Klapproth J-MA. Crohn's disease–associated Escherichia Coli survive in macrophages by suppressing NFκB signaling. Inflammatory Bowel Diseases. 2014;**20**:1419-1425. DOI: 10.1097/MIB.0000000000000096

[33] Tawfik A, Flanagan PK, Escherichia CBJ. Coli-host macrophage interactions in the pathogenesis of inflammatory bowel disease. World Journal of Gastroenterology. 2014;**20**:8751-8763. DOI: 10.3748/wjg.v20.i27.8751

[34] Weisshof R, Chermesh I. Micronutrient deficiencies in inflammatory bowel disease. Current Opinion in Clinical Nutrition and Metabolic Care. 2015;**18**:576-581. DOI: 10.1097/MCO.0000000000000226

[35] Rocha R, Santana GO, Almeida N, Lyra AC. Analysis of fat and muscle mass in patients with inflammatory bowel disease during remission and active phase. The British Journal of Nutrition. 2009;**101**:676-679. DOI: 10.1017/S0007114508032224

[36] Wiskin AE, Wootton SA, Hunt TM, Cornelius VR, Afzal NA, Jackson AA, et al. Body composition in childhood inflammatory bowel disease. Clinical Nutrition. 2011;**30**:112-115. DOI: 10.1016/j.clnu.2010.07.014

[37] Scaldaferri F, Pizzoferrato M, Lopetuso LR, Musca T, Ingravalle F, Sicignano LL, et al. Nutrition and IBD: Malnutrition and/or sarcopenia? A practical guide. Gastroenterology Research and Practice. 2017;**2017**. DOI: 10.1155/2017/8646495

[38] Hebuterne X, Filippi J, Al-Jaouni R, Nutritional SS. Consequences and nutrition therapy in Crohn's disease. Gastroentérologie Clinique et Biologique. 2009;**33**(Suppl 3):S235-S244. DOI: 10.1016/S0399-8320(09)73159-8

[39] Lucendo AJ, De Rezende LC. Importance of nutrition in inflammatory bowel disease. World Journal of Gastroenterology. 2009;**15**:2081-2088. DOI: 10.3748/wjg.15.2081

[40] Urbano APS, Sassaki LY, Dorna MS, Carvalhaes MA de BL, Martini LA, Ferreira ALA. Nutritional intake according to injury extent in ulcerative colitis patients. Journal of Human Nutrition and Dietetics. 2013;**26**:445-451. DOI: 10.1111/jhn.12064

[41] Ghishan FK, Epithelial KPR. Transport in inflammatory bowel diseases. Inflammatory Bowel Diseases. 2014;**20**:1099-1109. DOI: 10.1097/MIB.0000000000000029

[42] Hwang C, Ross V, Mahadevan U. Micronutrient deficiencies in inflammatory bowel disease: From a to zinc. Inflammatory Bowel Diseases. 2012;**18**:1961-1981. DOI: 10.1002/ibd.22906

[43] Capristo E, Addolorato G, Mingrone G, Greco AV, Gasbarrini G. Effect of disease localization on the anthropometric and metabolic features of Crohn's disease. The American Journal of Gastroenterology. 1998;**93**:2411-2419. DOI: 10.1111/j.1572-0241.1998.00696.x

[44] Santilli V, Bernetti A, Mangone M, Clinical PM. Definition of sarcopenia. Clinical Cases in Mineral and Bone Metabolism. 2014;**11**:177-180

[45] Bryant RV, Trott MJ, Bartholomeusz FD, Andrews JM. Systematic review: Body composition in adults with inflammatory bowel disease. Alimentary Pharmacology & Therapeutics. 2013;**38**:213-225. DOI: 10.1111/apt.12372

[46] Flores A, Burstein E, Cipher DJ, Feagins LA. Obesity in inflammatory bowel disease: A marker of less severe disease. Digestive Diseases and Sciences. 2015;**60**:2436-2445. DOI: 10.1007/s10620-015-3629-5

[47] Seminerio JL, Koutroubakis IE, Ramos-Rivers C, Hashash JG, Dudekula A, Regueiro M, et al. Impact of obesity on the management and clinical course of patients with inflammatory bowel disease. Inflammatory Bowel Diseases. 2015;**21**:2857-2863. DOI: 10.1097/MIB.0000000000000560

[48] Dignass AU, Gasche C, Bettenworth D, Birgegard G, Danese S, Gisbert JP, et al. European consensus on the diagnosis and management of iron deficiency and anaemia in inflammatory bowel diseases. Journal of Crohn's & Colitis. 2015;**9**:211-222. DOI: 10.1093/ecco-jcc/jju009

[49] Bermejo F, Algaba A, Guerra I, Chaparro M, De-La-Poza G, Valer P, et al. Should we monitor vitamin B12 and folate levels in Crohn's disease patients? Scandinavian Journal of Gastroenterology. 2013;**48**:1272-1277. DOI: 10.3109/00365521.2013.836752

[50] Yakut M, Ustun Y, Kabacam G, Soykan I. Serum vitamin B12 and folate status in patients with inflammatory bowel diseases. European Journal of Internal Medicine. 2010;**21**:320-323. DOI: 10.1016/j.ejim.2010.05.007

[51] Alves RA, Miszputen SJ, Figueiredo MS. Anemia in inflammatory bowel disease: Prevalence, differential diagnosis and association with clinical and laboratory variables. São Paulo Medical Journal. 2014;**132**:140-146

[52] Ananthakrishnan AN, Khalili H, Higuchi LM, Bao Y, Korzenik JR, Giovannucci EL, et al. Higher predicted vitamin D status is associated with reduced risk of Crohn's disease. Gastroenterology. 2012;**142**:482-489. DOI: 10.1053/j.gastro.2011.11.040

[53] Kong J, Zhang Z, Musch MW, Ning G, Sun J, Hart J, et al. Novel role of the vitamin D receptor in maintaining the integrity of the intestinal mucosal barrier. American Journal of Physiology. Gastrointestinal and Liver Physiology. 2008;**294**:G208-G216. DOI: 10.1152/ajpgi.00398.2007

[54] Levine A, Turner D, Pfeffer Gik T, Amil Dias J, Veres G, Shaoul R, et al. Comparison of outcomes parameters for induction of remission in new onset pediatric Crohn's disease. Inflammatory Bowel Diseases. 2014;**20**:278-285. DOI: 10.1097/01.MIB.0000437735.11953.68

[55] Lochs H, Forbes A. Nutritional Support in inflammatory bowel disease. In: Sobotka L, editor. Basics of Clinical Nutrition. 4th Ed., Prague: ESPEN. Publishing House Galen; 2011, p. 458-466

[56] Royall D, Greenberg GR, Allard JP, Baker JP, Harrison JE, Jeejeebhoy KN. Critical assessment of body-composition measurements in malnourished subjects with Crohn's disease: The role of bioelectric impedance analysis. The American Journal of Clinical Nutrition. 1994;**59**:325-330

[57] Vidarsdottir JB, Johannsdottir SE, Thorsdottir I, Bjornsson E, Ramel AA. Cross-sectional study on nutrient intake and -status in inflammatory bowel disease patients. Nutrition Journal. 2016;**15**:61. DOI: 10.1186/s12937-016-0178-5

[58] Ruemmele FMM, Veres G, Kolho KLL, Griffiths A, Levine A, Escher JCC, et al. Consensus guidelines of ECCO/ESPGHAN on the medical management of pediatric Crohn's disease. Journal of Crohn's & Colitis. 2014;**8**:1179-1207. DOI: 10.1016/j.crohns.2014.04.005

[59] Day AS, Lopez RN. Exclusive enteral nutrition in children with Crohn's disease. World Journal of Gastroenterology. 2015;**21**:6809-6816. DOI: 10.3748/wjg.v21.i22.6809

[60] Otley AR, Russell RK, Day AS. Nutritional therapy for the treatment of pediatric Crohn's disease. Expert Review of Clinical Immunology. 2010;**6**:667-676. DOI: 10.1586/eci.10.37

[61] Borrelli O, Cordischi L, Cirulli M, Paganelli M, Labalestra V, Uccini S, et al. Polymeric diet alone versus corticosteroids in the treatment of active pediatric Crohn's disease: A randomized controlled open-label trial. Clinical Gastroenterology and Hepatology. 2006;**4**:744-753. DOI: 10.1016/j.cgh.2006.03.010

[62] Zachos M, Tondeur M, Griffiths AM. Enteral nutritional therapy for induction of remission in Crohn's disease. In: Zachos M, editor. Cochrane Database of Systematic Reviews, Chichester, UK: John Wiley & Sons, Ltd; 2007, p. CD000542. DOI:10.1002/14651858. CD000542.pub2

[63] Yamamoto T, Nakahigashi M, Saniabadi AR. Review article : Diet and inflammatory bowel disease – Epidemiology and treatment. Alimentary Pharmacology & Therapeutics. 2009;**30**:99-112. DOI: 10.1111/j.1365-2036.2009.04035.x

[64] Malchow H, Steinhardt HJ, Lorenz-Meyer H, Strohm WD, Rasmussen S, Sommer H, et al. Feasibility and effectiveness of a defined-formula diet regimen in treating active Crohn's disease. European cooperative Crohn's disease study III. Scandinavian Journal of Gastroenterology. 1990;**25**:235-244

[65] Griffiths AM, Ohlsson A, Sherman PM, Sutherland LR. Meta-analysis of enteral nutrition as a primary treatment of active Crohn's disease. Gastroenterology. 1995;**108**:1056-1067

[66] Jackson CA, Clatworthy J, Robinson A, Horne R. Factors associated with non-adherence to oral medication for inflammatory bowel disease: A systematic review. The American Journal of Gastroenterology. 2010;**105**:525-539. DOI: 10.1038/ajg.2009.685

[67] Johnson T, Macdonald S, Hill SM, Thomas A, Murphy MS. Treatment of active Crohn's disease in children using partial enteral nutrition with liquid formula: A randomised controlled trial. Gut. 2006;**55**:356-361. DOI: 10.1136/gut.2004.062554

[68] Sigall-Boneh R, Pfeffer-Gik T, Segal I, Zangen T, Boaz M, Levine A. Partial enteral nutrition with a Crohn's disease exclusion diet is effective for induction of remission in children and young adults with Crohn's disease. Inflammatory Bowel Diseases. 2014;**20**:1353-1360. DOI: 10.1097/MIB.0000000000000110

[69] Gupta K, Noble A, Kachelries KE, Albenberg L, Kelsen JR, Grossman AB, et al. A novel enteral nutrition protocol for the treatment of pediatric Crohn's disease. Inflammatory Bowel Diseases. 2013;**19**:1374-1378

[70] Akobeng AK, Thomas AG. Enteral nutrition for maintenance of remission in Crohn's disease. In: Akobeng AK, editor. Cochrane Database of Systematic Reviews, Chichester, UK: John Wiley & Sons, Ltd; 2007, p. CD005984. DOI:10.1002/14651858.CD005984.pub2

[71] Nakahigashi M, Yamamoto T, Sacco R, Hanai H, Enteral KF. Nutrition for maintaining remission in patients with quiescent Crohn's disease: Current status and future perspectives. International Journal of Colorectal Disease. 2016;**31**:1-7. DOI: 10.1007/s00384-015-2348-x

[72] El-Matary W, Otley A, Critch J, Abou-Setta AM. Enteral feeding therapy for maintaining remission in Crohn's disease: A systematic review. Journal of Parenteral and Enteral Nutrition. 2017;**41**:550-561. DOI: 10.1177/0148607115621051

[73] Wilschanski M, Sherman P, Pencharz P, Davis L, Corey M, Griffiths A. Supplementary enteral nutrition maintains remission in paediatric Crohn's disease. Gut. 1996;**38**:543-548

[74] Scolapio JS. The role of total parenteral nutrition in the management of patients with acute attacks of inflammatory bowel disease. Journal of Clinical Gastroenterology. 1999;**29**:223-224

[75] Goh J, C a O'M. Nutrition and adult inflammatory bowel disease. Alimentary Pharmacology & Therapeutics. 2003;**17**:307-320. DOI: 10.1046/j.1365-2036.2003.01482.x

[76] Richman E, Rhodes JM. Review article: Evidence-based dietary advice for patients with inflammatory bowel disease. Alimentary Pharmacology & Therapeutics. 2013;**38**:1156-1171. DOI: 10.1111/apt.12500

[77] Forbes A, Escher J, Hebuterne X, Klek S, Krznaric Z, Schneider S, et al. ESPEN guideline: Clinical nutrition in inflammatory bowel disease. Clinical Nutrition. 2017;**36**:321-347. DOI: 10.1016/j.clnu.2016.12.027

[78] Owczarek D, Rodacki T, Domagała-rodacka R, Cibor D, Mach T, Owczarek D, et al. Diet and nutritional factors in inflammatory bowel diseases. World Journal of Gastroenterology. 2016;**22**:895-905. DOI: 10.3748/wjg.v22.i3.895

[79] Vanhauwaert E, Matthys C, Verdonck L, De Preter V. Low-residue and low-fiber diets in gastrointestinal disease management. Advances in Nutrition: An International Review Journal. 2015;**6**:820-827. DOI: 10.3945/an.115.009688

[80] Levenstein S, Prantera C, Luzi C, D'Ubaldi A. Low residue or normal diet in Crohn's disease: A prospective controlled study in Italian patients. Gut. 1985;**26**:989-993. DOI: 10.1136/gut.26.10.989

[81] Hoekman DR, Zeevenhooven J, D'Haens GR, Benninga MA. The prevalence of irritable bowel syndrome-type symptoms in inflammatory bowel disease patients in remission. European Journal of Gastroenterology & Hepatology. 2017;**29**:1086-1090. DOI: 10.1097/MEG.0000000000000921

[82] Prince AC, Myers CE, Joyce T, Irving P, Lomer M, Whelan K. Fermentable carbohydrate restriction (low FODMAP diet) in clinical practice improves functional gastrointestinal symptoms in patients with inflammatory bowel disease. Inflammatory Bowel Diseases. 2016;**22**:1129-1136. DOI: 10.1097/MIB.0000000000000708

[83] Brotherton CS, Taylor AG, Bourguignon C, Anderson JG. A high-fiber diet may improve bowel function and health-related quality of life in patients with Crohn disease. Gastroenterology Nursing. 2014;**37**:206-216. DOI: 10.1097/SGA.0000000000000047

[84] Hallert C, Bjorck I, Nyman M, Pousette A, Granno C, Svensson H. Increasing fecal butyrate in ulcerative colitis patients by diet: Controlled pilot study. Inflammatory Bowel Diseases. 2003;**9**:116-121

[85] Hallert C, Kaldma M, Petersson BG. Ispaghula husk may relieve gastrointestinal symptoms in ulcerative colitis in remission. Scandinavian Journal of Gastroenterology. 1991;**26**:747-750. DOI: 10.3109/00365529108998594

[86] Fernandez-Banares F, Hinojosa J, Sanchez-Lombrana JL, Navarro E, Martinez-Salmeron JF, Garcia-Puges A, et al. Randomized clinical trial of Plantago Ovata seeds (dietary fiber) as compared with mesalamine in maintaining remission in ulcerative colitis. Spanish Group for the Study of Crohn's Disease and Ulcerative Colitis (GETECCU). The American Journal of Gastroenterology. 1999;**94**:427-433. DOI: 10.1111/j.1572-0241.1999.872_a.x

[87] Hanai H, Kanauchi O, Mitsuyama K, Andoh A, Takeuchi K, Takayuki I, et al. Germinated barley foodstuff prolongs remission in patients with ulcerative colitis. International Journal of Molecular Medicine. 2004;**13**:643-647

[88] Faghfoori Z, Shakerhosseini R, Navai L, Somi MH, Nikniaz Z, Abadi A. Effects of an oral supplementation of germinated barley foodstuff on serum CRP level and clinical signs in patients with ulcerative colitis. Health Promotion Perspectives. 2014;**4**:116-121. DOI: 10.5681/hpp.2014.015

[89] Faghfoori Z, Navai L, Shakerhosseini R, Somi MH, Nikniaz Z, Norouzi MF. Effects of an oral supplementation of germinated barley foodstuff on serum tumour necrosis factor-alpha, interleukin-6 and -8 in patients with ulcerative colitis. Annals of Clinical Biochemistry. 2011;**48**:233-237. DOI: 10.1258/acb.2010.010093

[90] Haas S. The value of the banana in the treatment of celiac disease. American Journal of Diseases of Children. 1924;**28**:421-437

[91] Cohen SA, Gold BD, Oliva S, Lewis J, Stallworth A, Koch B, et al. Clinical and mucosal improvement with specific carbohydrate diet in pediatric Crohn disease. Journal of Pediatric Gastroenterology and Nutrition. 2014;**59**:516-521. DOI: 10.1097/MPG.0000000000000449

[92] Has S, Haas M. The treatment of celiac disease with the specific carbohydrate diet; report on 191 additional cases. The American Journal of Gastroenterology. 1955;**23**:344-360

[93] Suskind DL, Wahbeh G, Gregory N, Vendettuoli H, Christie D. Nutritional therapy in pediatric Crohn disease: The specific carbohydrate diet. Journal of Pediatric Gastroenterology and Nutrition. 2014;**58**:87-91. DOI: 10.1097/MPG.0000000000000103

[94] Wahbeh GT, Ward BT, Lee DY, Giefer MJ, Suskind DL. Lack of mucosal healing from modified specific carbohydrate diet in pediatric patients with Crohn disease. Journal of Pediatric Gastroenterology and Nutrition. 2017;**65**:289-292. DOI: 10.1097/MPG.0000000000001619

[95] Olendzki BC, Silverstein TD, Persuitte GM, Ma Y, Baldwin KR, An CD. Anti-inflammatory diet as treatment for inflammatory bowel disease: A case series report. Nutrition Journal. 2014;**13**:1-7. DOI: 10.1186/1475-2891-13-5

[96] Bao X, Feng Z, Yao J, Li T, Yin Y. Roles Of dietary amino acids and their metabolites in pathogenesis of inflammatory bowel disease. Mediators of Inflammation. 2017;2017:6869259. DOI:10.1155/2017/6869259

[97] Barbalho SM. Goulart R de a, Quesada K, Bechara MD, de Carvalho a de CA. Inflammatory bowel disease: Can omega-3 fatty acids really help? Ann Gastroenterol Q Publ Hell Soc Gastroenterol. 2016;**29**:37-43

[98] Meeker S, Seamons A, Maggio-Price L, Paik J. Protective links between vitamin D, inflammatory bowel disease and colon cancer. World Journal of Gastroenterology. 2016;**22**:933-948. DOI: 10.3748/wjg.v22.i3.933

[99] Vecchi Brumatti L, Marcuzzi A, Tricarico PM, Zanin V, Girardelli M, Bianco AM. Curcumin and inflammatory bowel disease: Potential and limits of innovative treatments. Molecules. 2014;**19**:21127-21153. DOI: 10.3390/molecules191221127

[100] Coëffier M, Marion-Letellier R, Potential DP. For amino acids supplementation during inflammatory bowel diseases. Inflammatory Bowel Diseases. 2010;**16**:518-524. DOI: 10.1002/ibd.21017

[101] Andou A, Hisamatsu T, Okamoto S, Chinen H, Kamada N, Kobayashi T, et al. Dietary histidine ameliorates murine colitis by inhibition of proinflammatory cytokine production from macrophages. Gastroenterology. 2009;**136**:564-74.e2. DOI:10.1053/j.gastro.2008.09.062

[102] Lee D, Albenberg L, Compher C, Baldassano R, Piccoli D, Lewis JD, et al. HHS public. Access. 2016;**148**:1087-1106. DOI: 10.1053/j.gastro.2015.01.007.Diet

[103] Kim CJ, Kovacs-Nolan JA, Yang C, Archbold T, Fan MZ, Mine Y. L-tryptophan exhibits therapeutic function in a porcine model of dextran sodium sulfate (DSS)-induced colitis. The Journal of Nutritional Biochemistry. 2010;**21**:468-475. DOI: 10.1016/j.jnutbio.2009.01.019

[104] Turner D, Zlotkin S, Shah P, Griffiths A. Omega 3 fatty acids (fish oil) for maintenance of remission in Crohn's disease. In: Turner D, editor. Cochrane Database of Systematic Reviews, Chichester, UK: John Wiley & Sons, Ltd; 2007, p. CD006320. DOI:10.1002/14651858.CD006320.pub2

[105] Meckel K, Li YC, Lim J, Kocherginsky M, Weber C, Almoghrabi A, et al. Serum 25-hydroxyvitamin D concentration is inversely associated with mucosal inflammation in patients with ulcerative colitis. The American Journal of Clinical Nutrition. 2016;**104**:113-120. DOI: 10.3945/ajcn.115.123786

[106] Raftery T, Merrick M, Healy M, Mahmud N, O'Morain C, Smith S, et al. Vitamin D status is associated with intestinal inflammation as measured by fecal calprotectin in Crohn's disease in clinical remission. Digestive Diseases and Sciences. 2015;**60**:2427-2435. DOI: 10.1007/s10620-015-3620-1

[107] Jorgensen SP, Agnholt J, Glerup H, Lyhne S, Villadsen GE, Hvas CL, et al. Clinical trial: Vitamin D3 treatment in Crohn's disease - A randomized double-blind placebo-controlled study. Alimentary Pharmacology & Therapeutics. 2010;**32**:377-383. DOI: 10.1111/j.1365-2036.2010.04355.x

[108] Kumar S, Ahuja V, Sankar MJ, Kumar A, Moss AC. Curcumin For maintenance of remission in ulcerative colitis. Cochrane Database of Systematic Reviews. 2012;**10**:CD008424. DOI:10.1002/14651858.CD008424.pub2

[109] Taylor RA, Curcumin LMC. For inflammatory bowel disease: A review of human studies. Alternative Medicine Review. 2011;**16**:152-156

Chapter 5

Exclusive and Partial Enteral Nutrition in Crohn's Disease

Darja Urlep, Evgen Benedik and Rok Orel

Additional information is available at the end of the chapter

http://dx.doi.org/10.5772/intechopen.72734

Abstract

Exclusive enteral nutrition (EEN) is a well-establised primary therapy in active pediatric Crohn's disease (CD). EEN promotes mucosal healing, restores bone mineral density, and improves growth. On the contrary, treatment of active CD with corticosteroids (CS) has a strong negative impact on the linear growth and bone density. Therefore, EEN is recommended as a first-line therapy in children with active CD. EEN has been evaluated in a number of clinical studies including randomized controlled trials. While meta-analyses of adult studies suggest superiority of CS, pediatric studies have shown that EEN is at least as effective as CS in inducing remission. The mechanisms by which EEN suppresses inflammation are not yet fully elucidated. Hypotheses include improvement in nutritional status, decreasing of the inflammatory cascade mechanism, limiting luminal antigen exposure, improving intestinal permeability, and modification of intestinal microbiota.

Keywords: Crohn's disease, exclusive enteral nutrition, partial enteral nutrition, children, adults

1. Introduction

Inflammatory bowel disease (IBD) is an immune-mediated condition, which includes Crohn's disease (CD), ulcerative colitis (UC), and IBD-unclassified (IBD-U) [1]. Nearly 25% of patients are diagnosed before 16 years of age. A number of studies have shown that pediatric-onset IBD presents with a more difficult phenotype when compared to adult-onset IBD and may have the consequences of growth retardation and delayed puberty as well as the psychological consequences of disease onset at a very vulnerable time of psychosocial development [2–5].

Exclusive enteral nutrition (EEN) is successful in the treatment of undernutrition. Moreover, EEN is able to induce remission in CD patients with active inflammation. The European Society of Gastroenterology, Hepatology and Nutrition (ESPGHAN) and the European Crohn's Colitis Organization (ECCO) recommend EEN as a first-line therapy in children with active CD and emphasize the use of EEN over CS in all children with active inflammatory intestinal luminal disease, including colonic involvement [6].

The therapy with EEN provides all of the nutritional needs by a liquid formula either orally or through a nasogastric tube. EEN is usually recommended for 6–8 weeks, and after this period, a normal diet is gradually reintroduced. For EEN therapy, elemental, semi-elemental, or polymeric formulas may be used. Elemental formulas are based on amino acids and contain no whole proteins, while semi-elemental formulas do contain peptides of varying lengths. Polymeric formulas are based on whole proteins and are therefore more palatable [7]. In addition, polymeric formulas usually cost less. The choice of formula most frequently depends on the clinician's experience and local availability [8].

EEN is especially recommended in CD children with stunted growth and in those presenting with low weight and a catabolic state. If EEN is not tolerated orally, a nasogastric tube may be used [6].

Nevertheless, EEN therapy remains underused in clinical practice, especially in adults in whom its efficacy in achieving clinical remission is considered to be less than the standard anti-inflammatory therapies [9].

In current review, different aspects of EEN as well as partial enteral nutrition (PEN) will be addressed, including their efficacy, treatment modalities, impact on mucosal healing, mechanisms of anti-inflammatory effects, and the role of enteral nutrition in maintaining remission.

2. The history of exclusive enteral nutrition

The first report on successful use of enteral feeding was published in 1973 by Voitk et al. It demonstrated improvement in inflammatory indices and weight gain in 13 patients. Nine of them were planned for surgery and two of them were able to avoid it after a period of exclusive elemental formula treatment [10].

In 1981, Logan et al. found a decrease in the number of gut lymphocytes and diminished protein loss when elemental enteral nutrition was used in patients with extensive small bowel CD [11].

Navarro et al. studied the efficacy of continuous elemental EEN on 17 pediatric patients with active CD and demonstrated that EEN was successful in inducing clinical remission. Additionally, therapy with EEN was proven to be safe and well tolerated [12].

Five years later, O'Morain et al. found that elemental EEN was equally successful or even more effective than steroids in inducing clinical remission in adults with active CD [13]. However, in 1995, a meta-analysis by Griffiths et al. demonstrated that therapy with EEN was significantly less effective compared to CS in a mixed population of adult and pediatric patients with CD [14]. But in 1997, in a randomized controlled trial by Zoli et al., EEN with an elemental diet was again shown to be equally effective as CS in inducing remission in a cohort of adult patients with both mild and moderately active CD [15].

3. Elemental versus polymeric enteral feeds

In the 1990s, both elemental and polymeric enteral nutrition were used in the largest pediatric inflammatory centers in United Kingdom as a first line of treatment of active CD. Clinical studies were then conducted to compare elemental versus polymeric enteral formulas [16]. In a randomized controlled trial by Rigaud et al., no significant difference was found in inducing clinical remission in adult CD patients between elemental and polymeric enteral formulas [17]. Ludvigsson et al. conducted a multicentre randomized control trial to compare the efficacy of elemental and polymeric formulas in children with active CD. The efficacy in inducing remission was found not to be different between elemental (E028E; Nutricia) and polymeric formulas (Nutrison Standard; Nutricia). However, patients who were receiving polymeric formula had better weight gain [18].

In a meta-analysis by Griffits et al., the efficacy of EEN therapy with elemental versus nonelemental formulas was compared. They demonstrated that there was no significant difference in the efficacy between the elemental and nonelemental formulas [14].

4. The efficacy of exclusive enteral nutrition versus corticosteroids

EEN has been evaluated in a number of clinical studies including randomized controlled trials (RCTs) that compared EEN with CS in adult and pediatric populations of patients with active CD. To date, eight meta-analyses have been published on the efficacy of EEN versus CS. Among these meta-analyses, three of them were performed exclusively on the pediatric population, whereas others included adult patients as well. While meta-analyses of adult studies have suggested better efficacy of CS, pediatric studies have shown that EEN is at least as effective as CS in inducing remission and is superior to CS in improving nutritional status and growth recovery without adverse side effects [19].

4.1. Efficacy of EEN versus CS in adult and mixed population of CD patients

In the first meta-analysis by Fernandez-Banares et al., the therapy with EEN was significantly less effective compared to CS. The meta-analysis included nine trials with mostly adult CD populations. The overall remission rate was 57.7% for EEN and 79.4% for CS [20]. A meta-analysis by Messori et al. included studies exclusively on the adult CD population which compared the effectiveness of EEN versus CS. The patient-specific end-point of the meta-analysis was occurrence of treatment failure. CS were more effective than EEN for inducing remission in adult active CD. In fact, the relative risk of treatment failure (RTF) was significantly lower in the steroid group than in the EEN group. They concluded that the data examined in this meta-analysis do not support the use of EEN as primary treatment for acute exacerbations of CD in adults [21]. In 1995, Griffiths et al. included eight RCTs (mixed adult and pediatric CD of 413 patients) comparing EEN with CS. Odds ratios (OR) for likelihood of clinical response were calculated. They found that EEN was inferior to CS (OR 0.35; 95% CI 0.23–0.53) [14]. A similar meta-analysis was performed in 2001 by the same team of authors from Toronto. In accordance with the stricter inclusion criteria, only four RCTs were included (130 patients treated with EEN and 123 treated with CS). The meta-analysis yielded a pooled OR for remission of 0.30 favoring CS therapy (95% CI 0.17–0.52) [22]. This meta-analysis was updated in 2007 and included six clinical trials with 192 patients treated with EEN and 160 treated with CS. The pooled OR for remission, after combining all type of enteral diets and comparing them with CS therapy, was 0.33 favoring steroid therapy (95% CI: 0.21–0.53) [23].

4.2. Efficacy of EEN versus CS in pediatric CD population

The first meta-analysis on pediatric population was published in 2000 by Heuschkel et al. The meta-analysis included five RCTs and was composed of 147 pediatric patients with active CD, and it demonstrated that EEN was equally effective as CS in inducing remission (relative risk (RR) = 0.95; 95% CI: 0.67–1.34). EEN was, however, superior in improving growth and pubertal development. Additionally, EEN seemed to be without the side effects. According to the results of this meta-analysis, EEN was then recommended as a first-line therapy in children with active CD [24]. The same results were demonstrated 7 years later in a meta-analysis by Dziechciarz et al. Only four RCTs (144 pediatric CD patients) met the inclusion criteria. No significant difference in remission rates between the patients receiving EEN and CS was found [25].

In the most recent published meta-analysis by Swaminath et al., eight clinical studies (451 pediatric CD patients) were included based on the inclusion criteria and availability of data that could be abstracted into meta-analysis. The efficacy in inducing remission was not different between EEN and CS (OR = 1.26; 95% CI 0.77–2.05). The authors also compared the efficacy between EEN and CS treatment in newly diagnosed CD patients (OR = 1.61; 95% CI 0.87–2.98) with relapsed patients (OR = 0.76; 95% CI 0.29–1.98) [26].

5. Recommendations on exclusive enteral nutrition in adult patients with Crohn's disease

To date, according to the results of meta-analyses on the adult CD population, EEN appears to be less effective than CS. Therefore, therapy with EEN is used as a first-line treatment in active CD only when therapy with CS is contraindicated [27].

In the current ECCO consensus guidelines for medical management of adult CD, therapy with enteral nutrition is regarded as a complementary treatment to improve nutrition and not as a primary therapy. It is still considered appropriate to use EEN in patients who decline all other drug therapies [28]. Further studies on EEN use as a primary therapy to induce remission in adult CD patients are needed to clarify the efficacy of EEN. The reasons for the difference in the efficacy of EEN between the pediatric and adult CD population have still not been elucidated. In adult IBD patients, who have a longer disease course and more frequent complications, EEN may be less effective. EEN may not be so strictly adhered to in adult patients, when compared to children, who are supervised by their parents. Furthermore, children and especially adolescents are generally more motivated to achieve success through this therapy. Most of them refuse CS treatment due to the unpleasant side effects related to appearance such as facies lunata, acne vulgaris, and increased hairiness.

6. Exclusive enteral nutrition and mucosal healing

Mucosal healing is an important therapeutic endpoint that, when achieved early, is associated with fewer hospitalizations, reduced surgical resections, lower risk of fistulizing disease, and less use of biologic drugs [29–32]. It is well established that treatment with EEN is capable of achieving mucosal healing in CD. On the contrary, CS have poor ability to induce mucosal healing. A study made in 1990, on the effects of prednisolone on mucosal healing in patients with active CD, found that 27% of patients still had minor lesions and only 12% achieved complete mucosal healing after 4–7 weeks of CS therapy [33]. Similarly, none out of eight patients with CD, treated with prednisolone for postoperative recurrence, showed mucosal healing after 6–9 weeks, based on the overall endoscopic assessment of the mucosa rather than a detailed endoscopic score [34]. These findings suggest that CS have little or no positive effects on induction of mucosal healing in CD. In a RCT in children with active CD, Borrelli et al. compared not only the efficacy of EEN versus CS in inducing clinical remission but also in achieving mucosal healing. The therapy with EEN was superior in achieving mucosal healing compared to CS. Mucosal healing was found in 14 of 19 CD patients (74%) in the EEN group and in 6 of 18 patients in the CS group (33%, $p < 0.05$) [35]. In a retrospective study by Berni Canani et al., 65% of pediatric CD patients on EEN therapy and 40% on CS ($p < 0.05$) achieved improvement in mucosal inflammation. Seven patients on EEN and none on CS were found to have complete mucosal healing ($p < 0.005$) at the end of treatment. In addition, the duration of clinical remission was longer in the EEN group when compared with the CS group [36]. Recently, Grover et al. had used the Simple Endoscopic Score for CD (SES-CD) to define endoscopic mucosal lesions in 26 children with active CD receiving EEN for 8 weeks. At the end of the EEN therapy, 42% of patients had complete mucosal healing (SES-CD = 0) and the other 58% had complete or near-complete mucosal healing (SES-CD < 3) [37]. Mucosal healing after EEN therapy was also demonstrated in the adult population of active CD patients. In a study by Yamamoto et al., a 4-week therapy with EEN has shown a complete endoscopic remission rate of 44% in the terminal ileum and 39% in the colon [38]. In a recent pediatric meta-analysis by Swaminath et al., two pediatric studies provided data on mucosal healing at the end of induction therapy with EEN versus CS [35, 36]. The occurrence of mucosal healing was significantly more likely in the group of CD children, who were receiving EEN, compared to those receiving CS (OR = 4.5; 95% CI 1.64–12.32) [26]. Furthermore, Rubio et al. compared fractionated oral versus continuous enteral feeding in terms of clinical and mucosal healing and have demonstrated similar rates of mucosal healing in patients receiving ether fractionated or continuous enteral feeding [39].

7. Disease location and efficacy of exclusive enteral nutrition

In the early 2000s, EEN was especially used in CD patients with small bowel disease. That was in accordance with the results of a clinical trial by Afzal et al. which have shown that EEN was less effective in CD patients with colonic disease in comparison with those who had only small bowel involvement or small and large bowel disease [40]. However, recent studies and meta-analyses have not confirmed this negative association [23, 25]. Buchanan et al. found no significant differences in remission rates in terms of disease location [41]. Similar findings were reported in a study by Rubio et al. where the site of disease activity had no impact on response to nutritional therapy [39]. The same results were demonstrated in a study by Gupta et al. where the location of the inflammation in CD did not affect the efficacy of EEN [42].

8. The long-term efficacy of exclusive enteral nutrition

The long-term efficacy of the induction therapy with EEN is not yet well established. Studies comparing the long-term outcomes of EEN versus CS treatment are limited. In a retrospective study by Lambert et al., a lower 1-year (61 versus 77%) and 2-year relapse rate (61 versus 89%) was demonstrated in CD children who were treated with EEN in comparison with those receiving CS [43]. Grover et al. have shown that induction therapy with EEN was superior to CS in reducing growth failure, CS dependency, and loss of response to infliximab over the first 2 years [44]. In a retrospective German study, most of the pediatric patients with active CD, treated with EEN, relapsed during the first year. Fortunately, 66% of them responded to a second course of EEN with remission [45]. In a recent study by Connors et al., both short- and long-term outcomes of EEN and CS induction therapy were examined. Out of 127 patients reviewed, a total of 111 propensity score-matched CD patients receiving EEN (n = 76) or CS (n = 35) were analyzed. Their data showed that clinical remission after EEN was superior to that after CS treatment, with 86.6 versus 58.1% of patients reaching remission within 4–12 weeks of starting treatment. This study supports a more optimistic view toward EEN as an approach to CS avoidance: over 40% of EEN-treated patients in their cohort remained steroid naive for at least 4 years. In addition, patients treated with EEN exhibited significantly greater improvement in height z-scores than patients treated with CS, at 1-year follow-up. The therapy with EEN over CS for induction of remission was associated with avoidance of CS over a 6-year follow-up period. This study showed that long-term steroid avoidance via EEN therapy is feasible without an increased need for escalation to anti-tumor necrosis factor alpha (anti-TNF-α). Most of the patients in the EEN-treated group who remained steroid-naive for 2 and 4 years had also not been exposed to anti-TNF-α, indicating that early anti-TNF-α use could account for only a minor portion of steroid avoidance in this group. They concluded that EEN induction therapy is more effective in achieving early remission and is associated with long-term steroid avoidance without increased use of biologics or need for surgery [46].

9. Current practice

Despite the reported benefits, EEN is not universally used in pediatric centers. Wide differences have been noted in the use of EEN between pediatric gastroenterologists in Europe and North America [47, 48]. A questionnaire-based study by Whitten et al. has shown wide variations in EEN protocols used in different areas of the world. Thirty-five centers were included in the study. The most centers recommend a 6–8 week therapy with polymeric formula and the gradual introduction of food quantity over 4–6 weeks [49].

10. The role of exclusive enteral nutrition in improvement of nutritional status and linear growth

Patients with IBD and especially children and adolescents often present with symptoms of undernutrition [50]. Both inflammation and undernutrition contribute to decreased height velocity [5]. Linear growth patterns correlate with disease activity, and there is strong pathophysiological evidence that inflammation interferes with the growth hormone axis [51, 52]. EEN decreases proinflammatory cytokines, including IL-6 and TNF-α, after which an increase in growth hormones (IGF-1 and IGFBP-3) is observed within 2 weeks of treatment [53]. It is not only that EEN decreases inflammation, it improves malnutrition and other specific nutritional deficiencies as well. Nutritional supplementation plays an important role in linear growth improvement. Importantly, EEN may also influence growth recovery in pediatric CD patients by limiting chronic corticosteroid exposure, which is a significant contributing factor toward growth failure [46, 54].

11. The role of preoperative exclusive enteral nutrition

To date, few experiences have been reported on the role of preoperative EEN in diminishing postoperative complications after bowel resections or other surgical interventions in patients with IBD. Li et al. investigated the influence of preoperative 3-month EEN on the incidence of postoperative intra-abdominal septic complications in CD patients with enterocutaneous fistulas. A retrospective study on 123 CD patients suffering from enterocutaneous fistulas was performed. The patients were divided into an EEN or a non-EEN group. A significantly lower rate of postoperative intra-abdominal septic complications was demonstrated in the EEN group versus the non-EEN group (3.6 versus 17.6%, $p < 0.05$). The results of this study have shown that preoperative EEN is an important factor for reduced risk of postoperative intra-abdominal septic complications [55]. The authors from the same IBD centre conducted another study to evaluate the impact of EEN on the perioperative outcome in CD patients following immunosuppressive therapy. There was a significant difference observed in the incidence of postoperative complications between the groups of CD patients who received and those who did not receive EEN ($p < 0.05$). In addition, the use of EEN decreased the need for urgent surgery and reoperation [56].

12. Mechanisms of action of exclusive enteral nutrition

Therapy with EEN substantially attenuates intestinal inflammation in CD patients. However, the mechanisms by which EEN suppresses inflammation are not yet fully understood. Hypotheses include improvement in nutritional intake and nutritional status, decreasing of the inflammatory cascade mechanism, limiting luminal antigen exposure, improving intestinal permeability, and modification of the intestinal microbiota [57]. Significant progress has been made in understanding mechanisms of how EEN suppresses inflammation. Basic research has demonstrated that EEN has direct anti-inflammatory properties, can correct localization of tight junction proteins and has other important impacts on intestinal permeability, alters micro RNAs expression, and profoundly affects the intestinal microbiota [58].

12.1. Anti-inflammatory effect of EEN

It is clear that EEN suppresses intestinal inflammation. In 1981, Logan et al. found a decrease in the number of gut lymphocytes and diminished protein loss when elemental enteral nutrition was used in patients with extensive small bowel CD [11]. In 1995, Breese et al. demonstrated that therapy with EEN reduced the number of lymphokine-secreting cells in the gut mucosa in CD [59]. Three years later, Beattie et al. reported on different mechanisms of action of EEN in CD. EEN was shown to be able to reduce the number of cytokine-producing cells in the inflamed mucosa of CD patients [16]. In a study by Fell et al., a decline in ileal and colonic interleukin-1beta mRNA was observed after 8 weeks of oral polymeric diet. In addition, a decrease of interferon gamma mRNA with a rise of transforming growth factor beta1 mRNA was demonstrated in the ileum and a fall of interleukin-8 mRNA in the colon [60]. Yamamoto et al. successfully managed acute duodenal CD with a low-speed elemental diet infusion via nasogastric tube in a 28-year-old female and also demonstrated that the duodenal mucosal cytokine levels remarkably decreased compared with those before the treatment [38]. Recently, Nahidi et al. cocultured heat tolerance (HT)-29 colonic epithelial cells with TNF-α in the presence or absence of polymeric formula, as used for EEN. Microarray analysis showed that polymeric formula modulated the expression of genes involved in the nuclear factor kB pathway with consequent downregulation of IL-6 and IL-8 proteins [61]. Alhagamhmad et al. wanted to find out whether the specific components in the polymeric formula drive the demonstrated attenuation of the nuclear factor kB cascade. They used tumor necrosis factor-α-exposed HT-29 colonic epithelial cells to investigate the immunosuppressive activity of the glutamine, arginine, vitamin D3, and α-linolenic acid (ALA), present in polymeric formula, along with curcumin. They found out that glutamine, arginine, and vitamin D3, but not ALA, significantly attenuated IL-8 production. Glutamine and arginine led to a phosphorylation blockade of the signaling components in NF-κB and P38 pathways, reduction in kinase activity, and enhancement in NO production. They concluded that glutamine, arginine, and vitamin D3 can suppress inflammation at concentrations equivalent to those used in polymeric formula. According to these findings, glutamine and arginine-fortified polymeric formulas might be a promising option to enhance the effectiveness of EEN therapy in CD treatment [57]. There is accumulating evidence that microRNAs play an important role in CD pathogenic processes, including regulation of pro and anti-inflammatory pathways. Guo et al. performed a microarray analysis in 25 adult CD patients and 10 healthy individuals treated with EEN. The microarray analysis showed that the mucosal micro RNAs expression profile is significantly altered after EEN therapy compared with the one in inflamed mucosa before EEN treatment [62]. The Australian investigators demonstrated that polymeric formula had a direct anti-inflammatory effect on colonic enterocytes. Polymeric formula was able to reduce interleukin (IL)-8 response to proinflammatory stimuli when it was added to the culture medium. The authors concluded that polymeric formula may modulate gut inflammation by directly reducing the inflammatory response of the intestinal epithelium [63]. Recently, the same team of investigators found that the incubation of human cells (Caco-2 human adenocarcinoma cell line) with a polymeric formula resulted in a dose-dependent increase in the expression of intestinal alkaline phosphatase, which is a recognized marker of enterocyte differentiation. Intestinal alkaline phosphatase is implicated in the innate gut immune response to enteric pathogens. This finding suggests that cell surface-associated intestinal alkaline phosphatase may be an aspect of the gut's innate immune response to pathogenic bacteria that is strengthened by polymeric formula [64].

12.2. Reduction in dietary antigen exposure

In the first years, only elemental formulas were used for the treatment of active CD. It was believed that the effect of EEN was based on exclusion of the dietary antigens which might have a role in inducing and promoting the inflammatory cascade. However, later research has shown that whole protein polymeric formulas were also as effective in inducing remission in patients with active CD [14, 18, 22, 65, 66].

12.3. The role of fats in EN formulas

The influence of the lipid source within the enteral feeds has been examined, but how the lipids composition of enteral nutrition affects its efficacy remains to be elucidated. In a meta-analysis by Zahos et al., the efficacy between the elemental formulas with low fat content (< 20 g/1000 kcal) versus high fat content (> 20 g/1000 kcal) was compared. This meta-analysis did not demonstrate a significant difference in efficacy of the two types of elemental formulas [23]. In the last decades, the impact of the use of fatty acids as potential immune-modulating agents in an inflammatory condition such as CD has been studied [67]. Recently, in a double-blind RCT by Grogan et al., a modest effect on the blood fatty acid composition was seen with both nutritional interventions (with Alicalm and Emsogen). After an intervention with a 6-week therapy with Alicalm, an increase of eicosapentaenoic acid (EPA) and alpha linolenic acid (ALA) was demonstrated with an inverse decrease in arachidonic acid (AA). Arachidonic acid is an important precursor to eicosanoids, which are second messengers in numerous signal transduction processes and have proinflammatory properties. The authors of this study concluded that there may be an advantage of using enteral formula that contains increased levels of ALA, as it is a precursor of anti-inflammatory eicosanoids [68].

12.4. Glutamin and arginine in EN formulas

Glutamine and arginine are conditionally essential amino acids with immunomodulatory properties. Glutamine may be essential in patients with catabolic conditions where the intervention with glutamine-supplements is able to prevent the deterioration of gut permeability and development of intestinal mucosal atrophy [69–71]. Akobeng et al. conducted a RCT, which included 18 pediatric patients with active CD, who were randomly assigned to receive a 4-week course of either: standard polymeric formula with low glutamine content (4% of amino acid composition) or a glutamine-enriched polymeric diet (42% of amino acid composition). They found no significant difference between these two types of formula in terms of clinical efficacy [72]. In a recent meta-analysis of the same authors, only two small RCTs (total 42 patients) met the inclusion criteria. The first study is the aforementioned pediatric study by Akobeng et al. [72]. In the second study, 24 adult CD patients with acute exacerbation of IBD were treated either with glutamine-supplemented or non-supplemented total parenteral nutrition. In both included studies, no statistically significant changes in intestinal permeability were found between patients, who received glutamine supplementation and those who did not [73]. Further randomized controlled clinical studies on the efficacy and safety of glutamin supplementation in patients with active CD are needed.

12.5. The impact of EEN on gut microbiota

While all the pathogenetic mechanisms of action of EEN have not yet been elucidated, EEN is known to cause profound changes in the gut microbiome. Understanding how EEN modifies the gut microbiome to induce remission could provide insight into CD etiopathogenesis and consequently guide the development of microbiome-targeted interventions [74]. In 2005, Lionetti et al. assessed clinical remission and the fecal microbiota in nine children with active CD treated with EEN. Clinical remission was observed in eight of nine children. In all these patients, significant modification of the fecal microbiota was found after EEN therapy. In contrast, control healthy children showed a host-specific and stable microbiota over time [75]. Similarly, Leach et al. demonstrated a significantly different composition of intestinal microbiota in patients with CD treated with EEN in comparison with the microbiota of control subjects. The effect of modificated microbiota remained present for 4 months after EEN [76]. EEN was shown to promote protective species and increase the production of butyrate [77]. Surprisingly, in a Scottish study which included 15 pediatric patients with CD before and after remission with EEN and 21 control subjects, the therapy with EEN was associated with a decrease in diversity of microbiota and not vice versa as was expected. A decrease in specific 'protective' species including *F. prausnitzii* was found as well as a fall in butyrate in fecal samples. These results have challenged the current perception of a protective role of *F. prausnitzii* in CD [78]. Quince et al. have analyzed microbiota in 23 CD children and in 21 healthy controls before, during, and after EEN treatment. They demonstrated lower microbial diversity in CD patients compared with controls before EEN. During the therapy with EEN, the microbial diversity in CD children further decreased and the structure of microbiota became even more dissimilar in comparison with the healthy controls [79]. In another small study, similar results were shown. Fecal microbiota of five children with CD, before, during, and after EEN treatment was analyzed and compared with five healthy controls. It showed a dramatic decrease in the number of operational taxonomic units (OTUs) after therapy with EEN. Inversely, recurrence of inflammation corresponded with an increase in OTUs [80]. In an extension study by Lee et al., fecal samples from patients (n = 86) treated with either PEN, EEN, or anti-TNF-α were analyzed using shotgun metagenomics analysis at four points of time during treatment and compared with healthy controls. After 1 week of treatment, the microbiota composition among the EEN-treated group drifted significantly farther from centroid of the healthy controls compared to anti-TNF-α treated patients who moved closer to the centroid. However, at the end of the study, responders (those with clinical remission and reduction in fecal calprotectin) were closer to the centroid of the healthy controls than nonresponders, regardless of treatment, suggesting that at treatment initiation, the treatment modality is the major determinant affecting gut microbiota, whereas later on, the resolution of inflammation becomes the dominant factor. Still, the resolution of dysbiosis was not complete even among responders at 8 weeks [81].

12.6. Exclusion of specific dietary components

During the 6- to 8-week therapy with EEN, the patients with active CD should not eat any food, and their 100% daily caloric requirements are covered by liquid formula. Therefore, the therapy with EEN automatically involves exclusion of many common dietary components which might have a deleterious effect on the intestinal mucosa. The avoidance of these potentially harmful dietary components might present another potential anti-inflammatory mechanism of EEN [82].

13. Partial enteral nutrition for maintaining remission in Crohn's disease

There are some studies suggesting that nutritional supplementation with liquid formulas may prolong remission in patients with quiescent CD [83–85]. However, the efficacy of partial enteral nutrition (PEN) for maintaining remission in inactive CD has not yet been fully evaluated. On the contrary, the use of immunomodulators and biological medications for maintaining remission in CD is well established. The adverse events of these medications, such as the increased risk of infection and malignancy, have always been concerning [86, 87]. Therefore, we should aim for a safer maintenance regimen, especially in children. Maintenance enteral nutrition (MEN) could be an attractive option for maintaining remission of inactive CD, as it will eliminate serious adverse events associated with the use of immunosuppressive medications and biologics. In 1987, Jones et al. reported their experience with 77 (16–65 years) CD patients in clinical remission who tried to maintain remission by personalized food exclusion diets along with a supplementary elemental diet. Twenty six of 77 (33.7%) patients remained in remission for 2 years and 18 (23.4%) patients for at least 3 years [88]. In a study by Wilschanski et al., pediatric patients with active CD who were successfully treated with EEN were assessed retrospectively according to whether they continued supplementary enteral nutrition or not. Time to relapse and linear growth were compared between the two cohorts. Patients who continued nasogastric supplementary feeding ($n = 28$) after reintroduction of their otherwise normal diet remained in remission longer than those who discontinued nocturnal supplementation ($n = 19$) ($p < 0.02$). Furthermore, continued use of nasogastric supplements before completion of puberty was associated with improved linear growth [85]. In 2000, Verma et al. studied a series of 39 consecutive patients with CD in clinical remission over 12 months. Patients in group 1 ($n = 21$) received oral nutritional supplementation along with their normal diet and patients in group 2 ($n = 18$) had a normal unrestricted diet without the nutritional supplementation. Forty-eight percent of patients in group 1 remained in remission for 12 months compared to the 22% of patients in group 2 ($p < 0.0003$) [89]. In 2007, Akonbeng et al. conducted a systematic review on the efficacy of enteral nutrition for maintenance of remission in CD. Only two studies were included based on the inclusion criteria

[90]. In the first study, a significant lower relapse rate was found in CD patients who received half of their daily nutritional needs from an elemental formula and the remaining half by normal diet compared to patients who only received a normal diet [90]. In the second study, the comparison between elemental and polymeric formulas (providing between 35 and 50% of patients' caloric intake in addition to normal diet) was assessed in terms of maintenance of remission. Both type of formulas were equally effective in maintaining remission and allowing withdrawal of steroid therapy [91, 92]. Recently, Nakahigashi et al. have reviewed the efficacy of EN for the maintenance of remission in patients with quiescent CD. Seven prospective cohort studies were included and three of them were RCTs. In all studies, patients used EN as a supplement or as a nocturnal tube feeding in addition to their normal food. The maintained clinical remission rate at 1 year was significantly higher in patients treated with EN in four of the six studies [93]. Although some studies suggest that PEN may be helpful for the maintenance of remission in the pediatric population [84, 85], data on the long-term usage of PEN for remission maintenance in pediatric CD patients are still lacking. A recent retrospective study by Schulman et al. investigated the efficacy of PEN treatment in the maintenance of remission in the pediatric CD population. In their centre, this approach has been in practice for the last several years. They assessed 42 pediatric CD patients who entered clinical remission on 4–12 weeks of EEN and were maintained on PEN as a supplementary diet (50% of total calories obtained as polymeric formula). The control group consisted of patients who refused PEN. They found that the decrease in the disease activity was greater in the PEN group than in the control group, as was the total increase in body mass index between the time of diagnosis and 8 months after. Laboratory parameters, such as albumin and CRP, also showed better improvement in the PEN group than in the control group. Although PEN was able to maintain short remission in patients initially treated with EEN, most of the patients required concomitant medication at some point after PEN initiation. They conclude that PEN treatment was partially effective in maintaining remission in patients who were initially treated with EEN. To better assess the efficacy of PEN for maintaining remission in children with CD, further prospective studies are required. Recently, El-Matary et al. have published a systematic review on the efficacy of MEN in adult and pediatric patients with CD. Twelve studies (1169 patients, including 95 children) fulfilled the inclusion criteria. As the included studies were significantly heterogeneous, a meta-analysis was not performed. Eleven studies showed that EN was either better than or as effective as its comparator in maintaining remission in patients with inactive CD. Only one adult RCT ($n = 51$), with low risk of bias, compared EN with a regular diet and found a relapse rate of 34% in the EN group versus 64% in the control group ($p < 0.01$) after a mean follow-up of 11.9 months. The authors concluded that EN is more effective than a regular diet and as effective as some medications in maintaining remission for patients with inactive CD. Large, properly designed RCTs of sufficient duration are, however, still required to confirm this outcome regarding EN versus individual medications [94].

14. Partial enteral nutrition in the treatment of active Crohn's disease

In 2006, Jones et al. have published the first RCT on partial enteral nutrition (PEN). Fifty children with active CD (PCDAI >20) were randomly assigned in PEN or EEN group. Children in PEN group had obtained 50% of their caloric requirements from elemental formula and 50% from unrestricted diet, while children in EEN had received 100% of their energy requirements from elemental formula for 6 weeks. This study showed that the conventional treatment with EEN was associated with a significantly higher remission rate in comparison with PEN (42 versus 15%) [95]. The next study on the efficacy of PEN was conducted at The Children's Hospital of Philadelphia (CHOP). The authors retrospectively studied the efficacy of their CHOP protocol of PEN, which allowed patients to consume 10–20% of their daily caloric needs from a normal diet and 80–90% from enteral nutrition. In this study, a remission rate of 65% and response rate of 87% were demonstrated, which is comparable with the remission rate of EEN from literature. The authors concluded that the use of the CHOP protocol may increase compliance in the population of pediatric CD patients by improving quality of life [42]. Recently, Sigall-Boneh et al. treated 47 patients (34 children and 13 young adults) with early mild-to-moderate luminal CD with PEN. Their approach allowed patients to consume 50% of dietary calories from a polymeric formula and remaining calories from a special Crohn's disease exclusion diet (CDED). In the study, a clinical response and remission were achieved in 78.7 and 70.2% patients, respectively. Surprisingly, in six of seven patients who refused PEN and used only the specific exclusion diet for CD, clinical remission was observed. This study has shown for the first time that a combination of PEN with the exclusion diet was successful and led to high remission rates in early mild-to-moderate luminal CD, in children and young adults [96]. Furthermore, the findings of this study suggest that specific dietary products may play a role in the promotion of intestinal mucosal inflammation. The authors of this study hypothesize that the major mechanism leading to response to EEN used in children with active CD is exclusion of specific dietary factors which may have negative impact on the innate immune mechanisms of intestinal mucosa such as the mucous layer, intestinal permeability, or colonization and adherence with adherent-invasive *E. coli* (AIEC). They suggest that specific dietary components such as additives may impair the barrier function of the intestinal epithelium and allow adherence and invasion of nonpathogenic bacteria or bacterial antigens. Adherence of bacteria to the intestinal epithelium, penetration, and replication within epithelial cells, dendritic cells, and macrophages leads to continuous triggering of the adaptive immune system, resulting in inflammation [97]. According to the results of recent epidemiological and animal model studies, they developed CDED based on exclusion of dietary components hypothesized to affect the microbiome or intestinal permeability or other elements of innate immune system involved in CD pathogenesis [82, 97]. CDED is a structured diet that excludes animal fats, milk and dairy, gluten, and all processed and canned foods, which contain additives (especially emulsifiers and maltodextrin) [96]. Although the authors from CHOP and Israel did show that PEN may be effective in inducing the remission in active CD, this approach of treatment is not recommended according to the ESPGHAN/ECCO guidelines on the treatment of active CD in pediatric population [6]. Further studies on the efficacy of PEN are warranted to elucidate the efficacy of this treatment approach.

15. Conclusion

EEN is recommended as a first-line therapy for remission induction in pediatric luminal Crohn's disease. Despite the inconsistent evidence regarding long-term efficacy, EEN has an established advantage over corticosteroids with comparable clinical efficacy but superior mucosal healing effect as well as better safety profile. The exact mechanism by which EEN exerts its beneficial impact is still not established, particularly, whether exclusion of specific potentially harmful dietary components plays an important role. Nevertheless, accumulating evidence suggest a direct anti-inflammatory effect and an effect on the intestinal microbiota. The relationships between these effects and the specific triggers for the observed changes are yet to be elucidated.

Conflict of interest

The authors have no conflicts of interest.

Author details

Darja Urlep*, Evgen Benedik and Rok Orel

*Address all correspondence to: darja.urlep@kclj.si

University Children's Hospital, University Medical Centre Ljubljana, Ljubljana, Slovenia

References

[1] Conrad MA, Rosh JR. Pediatric inflammatory bowel disease. Pediatric Clinics of North America. 2017;**64**:577-591. DOI: 10.1016/j.pcl.2017.01.005

[2] Vernier–Massouille G, Balde M, Salleron J, Turck D, Dupas JL, Mouterde O, et al. Natural history of pediatric Crohn's disease: A population-based cohort study. Gastroenterology 2008;**135**:1106-1113. DOI: 10.1053/j.gastro.2008.06.079

[3] Van Limbergen J, Russell RK, Drummond HE, Aldhous MC, Round NK, Nimmo ER, et al. Definition of phenotypic characteristics of childhood-onset inflammatory bowel disease. Gastroenterology. 2008;**135**:1114-1122. DOI: 10.1053/j.gastro.2008.06.081

[4] Pigneur B, Seksik P, Viola S, Viala J, Beaugerie L, Girardet J-P, et al. Natural history of Crohn's disease. Inflammatory Bowel Diseases. 2010;**16**:953-961. DOI: 10.1002/ibd.21152

[5] Griffiths AM. Growth retardation in early-onset inflammatory bowel disease: Should we monitor and treat these patients differently? Digestive Diseases. 2009;**27**:404-411. DOI: 10.1159/000228581

[6] Ruemmele FM, Veres G, Kolho KL, Griffiths A, Levine A, Escher JC, et al. Consensus guidelines of ECCO/ESPGHAN on the medical management of pediatric Crohn's disease. Journal of Crohn's and Colitis. 2014;**8**:1179-1207. DOI: 10.1016/j.crohns.2014.04.005

[7] Malchow H, Steinhardt HJ, Lorenz-Meyer H, Strohm WD, Rasmussen S, Sommer H, et al. Feasibility and effectiveness of a defined-formula diet regimen in treating active Crohn's disease. European cooperative Crohn's disease study III. Scandinavian Journal of Gastroenterology 1990;**25**:235-244

[8] Critch J, Day AS, Otley A, King-Moore C, Teitelbaum JE, Shashidhar H, et al. Use of enteral nutrition for the control of intestinal inflammation in pediatric Crohn's disease. Journal of Pediatric Gastroenterology and Nutrition. 2012;**54**:298-305. DOI: 10.1097/MPG.0b013e318235b397

[9] Kansal S, Wagner J, Kirkwood CD, Catto-Smith AG. Enteral nutrition in Crohn's disease: An underused therapy. Gastroenterology Research and Practice. 2013;**2013**:1-11. DOI: 10.1155/2013/482108

[10] Voitk AJ, Echave V, Feller JH, Brown RA, Gurd FN. Experience with elemental diet in the treatment of inflammatory bowel disease. Is this primary therapy? Archives of Surgery 1973;**107**:329-333

[11] Logan RF, Gillon J, Ferrington C, Ferguson A. Reduction of gastrointestinal protein loss by elemental diet in Crohn's disease of the small bowel. Gut. 1981;**22**:383-387

[12] Navarro J, Vargas J, Cezard JP, Charritat JL, Polonovski C. Prolonged constant rate elemental enteral nutrition in Crohn's disease. Journal of Pediatric Gastroenterology and Nutrition. 1982;**1**:541-546

[13] O'Morain C. Elemental diets and Crohn's disease. Acta Gastroenterologica Belgica. 1987;**50**:574-578

[14] Griffiths AM, Ohlsson A, Sherman PM, Sutherland LR. Meta-analysis of enteral nutrition as a primary treatment of active Crohn's disease. Gastroenterology. 1995;**108**:1056-1067

[15] Zoli G, Carè M, Parazza M, Spanò C, Biagi PL, Bernardi M, et al. A randomized controlled study comparing elemental diet and steroid treatment in Crohn's disease. Alimentary Pharmacology & Therapeutics. 1997;**11**:735-740

[16] Beattie RM, Bentsen BS, MacDonald TT. Childhood Crohn's disease and the efficacy of enteral diets. Nutrition 1998;**14**:345-350

[17] Rigaud D, Cosnes J, Le Quintrec Y, René E, Gendre JP, Mignon M. Controlled trial comparing two types of enteral nutrition in treatment of active Crohn's disease: Elemental versus polymeric diet. Gut. 1991;**32**:1492-1497

[18] Ludvigsson JF, Krantz M, Bodin L, Stenhammar L, Lindquist B. Elemental versus polymeric enteral nutrition in paediatric Crohn's disease: A multicentre randomized controlled trial. Acta Paediatrica. 2004;**93**:327-335

[19] Levine A, Turner D, Pfeffer Gik T, Amil Dias J, Veres G, Shaoul R, et al. Comparison of outcomes parameters for induction of remission in new onset pediatric Crohn's disease. Inflammatory Bowel Diseases. 2014;**20**:278-285. DOI: 10.1097/01.MIB.0000437735.11953.68

[20] Fernández-Bañares F, Cabré E, Esteve-Comas M, Gassull MA. How effective is enteral nutrition in inducing clinical remission in active Crohn's disease? A meta-analysis of the randomized clinical trials. Journal of Parenteral and Enteral Nutrition. 1995;**19**:356-364. DOI: 10.1177/0148607195019005356

[21] Messori A, Trallori G, D'Albasio G, Milla M, Vannozzi G, Pacini F. Defined-formula diets versus steroids in the treatment of active Crohn's disease: A meta-analysis. Scandinavian Journal of Gastroenterology. 1996;**31**:267-272

[22] Zachos M, Tondeur M, Griffiths A. Enteral nutritional therapy for induction of remission in Crohn's disease. In: Zachos M, editor. Cochrane Database of Systematic Reviews. Chichester, UK: John Wiley & Sons, Ltd; 2001. p. CD000542. DOI: 10.1002/14651858.CD000542

[23] Zachos M, Tondeur M, Griffiths AM. Enteral nutritional therapy for induction of remission in Crohn's disease. In: Zachos M, editor. Cochrane Database of Systematic Reviews. Chichester, UK: John Wiley & Sons, Ltd; 2007. p. CD000542. DOI: 10.1002/14651858.CD000542.pub2

[24] Heuschkel RB, Menache CC, Megerian JT, Baird AE. Enteral nutrition and corticosteroids in the treatment of acute Crohn's disease in children. Journal of Pediatric Gastroenterology and Nutrition. 2000;**31**:8-15

[25] Dziechciarz P, Horvath A, Shamir R, Szajewska H. Meta-analysis: Enteral nutrition in active Crohn's disease in children. Alimentary Pharmacology & Therapeutics. 2007;**26**:795-806. DOI: 10.1111/j.1365-2036.2007.03431.x

[26] Swaminath A, Feathers A, Ananthakrishnan AN, Falzon L, Li Ferry S. Systematic review with meta-analysis: Enteral nutrition therapy for the induction of remission in paediatric Crohn's disease. Alimentary Pharmacology & Therapeutics. 2017;**46**:645-656. DOI: 10.1111/apt.14253

[27] Lochs H, Dejong C, Hammarqvist F, Hebuterne X, Leon-Sanz M, Schütz T, et al. ESPEN guidelines on enteral nutrition: Gastroenterology. Clinical Nutrition. 2006;**25**:260-274. DOI: 10.1016/j.clnu.2006.01.007

[28] Esser D, Cornillie F, Diamond RH, Spiegel RJ. On the updated ECCO consensus guidelines for medical management of Crohn's disease. Journal of Crohn's and Colitis. 2011;**5**:165-166. DOI: 10.1016/j.crohns.2010.02.002

[29] Baert F, Moortgat L, Van Assche G, Caenepeel P, Vergauwe P, De Vos M, et al. Mucosal healing predicts sustained clinical remission in patients with early-stage Crohn's disease. Gastroenterology. 2010;**138**:463-468. DOI: 10.1053/j.gastro.2009.09.056

[30] Schnitzler F, Fidder H, Ferrante M, Noman M, Arijs I, Van Assche G, et al. Mucosal healing predicts long-term outcome of maintenance therapy with infliximab in Crohn's disease. Inflammatory Bowel Diseases. 2009;**15**:1295-1301. DOI: 10.1002/ibd.20927

[31] D'Haens G, Baert F, van Assche G, Caenepeel P, Vergauwe P, Tuynman H, et al. Early combined immunosuppression or conventional management in patients with newly diagnosed Crohn's disease: An open randomised trial. Lancet. 2008;**371**:660-667. DOI: 10.1016/S0140-6736(08)60304-9

[32] Neurath MF, Travis SPL. Mucosal healing in inflammatory bowel diseases: A systematic review. Gut. 2012;**61**:1619-1635. DOI: 10.1136/gutjnl-2012-302830

[33] Modigliani R, Mary JY, Simon JF, Cortot A, Soule JC, Gendre JP, et al. Clinical, biological, and endoscopic picture of attacks of Crohn's disease. Evolution on prednisolone. Groupe d'Etude Thérapeutique des Affections Inflammatoires Digestives. Gastroenterology 1990;**98**:811-818

[34] Olaison G, Sjödahl R, Tagesson C. Glucocorticoid treatment in ileal Crohn's disease: Relief of symptoms but not of endoscopically viewed inflammation. Gut. 1990;**31**:325-328

[35] Borrelli O, Cordischi L, Cirulli M, Paganelli M, Labalestra V, Uccini S, et al. Polymeric diet alone versus corticosteroids in the treatment of active pediatric Crohn's disease: A randomized controlled open-label trial. Clinical Gastroenterology and Hepatology. 2006;**4**:744-753. DOI: 10.1016/j.cgh.2006.03.010

[36] Berni Canani R, Terrin G, Borrelli O, Romano MT, Manguso F, Coruzzo A, et al. Short- and long-term therapeutic efficacy of nutritional therapy and corticosteroids in paediatric Crohn's disease. Digestive and Liver Disease. 2006;**38**:381-387. DOI: 10.1016/j.dld.2005.10.005

[37] Grover Z, Muir R, Lewindon P. Exclusive enteral nutrition induces early clinical, mucosal and transmural remission in paediatric Crohn's disease. Journal of Gastroenterology. 2014;**49**:638-645. DOI: 10.1007/s00535-013-0815-0

[38] Yamamoto T, Nakahigashi M, Umegae S, Kitagawa T, Matsumoto K. Impact of elemental diet on mucosal inflammation in patients with active Crohn's disease: Cytokine production and endoscopic and histological findings. Inflammatory Bowel Diseases. 2005;**11**:580-588

[39] Rubio A, Pigneur B, Garnier-Lengliné H, Talbotec C, Schmitz J, Canioni D, et al. The efficacy of exclusive nutritional therapy in paediatric Crohn's disease, comparing fractionated oral vs. continuous enteral feeding. Alimentary Pharmacology & Therapeutics. 2011;**33**:1332-1339. DOI: 10.1111/j.1365-2036.2011.04662.x

[40] Afzal NA, Davies S, Paintin M, Arnaud-Battandier F, Walker-Smith JA, Murch S, et al. Colonic Crohn's disease in children does not respond well to treatment with enteral nutrition if the ileum is not involved. Digestive Diseases and Sciences. 2005;**50**:1471-1475

[41] Buchanan E, Gaunt WW, Cardigan T, Garrick V, McGrogan P, Russell RK. The use of exclusive enteral nutrition for induction of remission in children with Crohn's disease demonstrates that disease phenotype does not influence clinical remission. Alimentary Pharmacology & Therapeutics. 2009;**30**:501-507. DOI: 10.1111/j.1365-2036.2009.04067.x

[42] Gupta K, Noble A, Kachelries KE, Albenberg L, Kelsen JR, Grossman AB, et al. A novel enteral nutrition protocol for the treatment of pediatric Crohn's disease. Inflammatory Bowel Diseases. 2013;**19**:1374-1378. DOI: 10.1097/MIB.0b013e318281321b

[43] Lambert B, Lemberg DA, Leach ST, Day AS. Longer-term outcomes of nutritional management of Crohn's disease in children. Digestive Diseases and Sciences. 2012;**57**:2171-2177. DOI: 10.1007/s10620-012-2232-2

[44] Grover Z, Lewindon P. Two-year outcomes after exclusive enteral nutrition induction are superior to corticosteroids in Pediatric Crohn's disease treated early with Thiopurines. Digestive Diseases and Sciences. 2015;**60**:3069-3074. DOI: 10.1007/s10620-015-3722-9

[45] Frivolt K, Schwerd T, Werkstetter KJ, Schwarzer A, Schatz SB, Bufler P, et al. Repeated exclusive enteral nutrition in the treatment of paediatric Crohn's disease: Predictors of efficacy and outcome. Alimentary Pharmacology & Therapeutics. 2014;**39**:1398-1407. DOI: 10.1111/apt.12770

[46] Connors J, Basseri S, Grant A, Giffin N, Mahdi G, Noble A, et al. Exclusive enteral nutrition therapy in paediatric Crohn's disease results in long-term avoidance of corticosteroids: Results of a propensity-score matched cohort analysis. Journal of Crohn's and Colitis. 2017;**11**:1063-1070. DOI: 10.1093/ecco-jcc/jjx060

[47] Van Limbergen J, Haskett J, Griffiths AM, Critch J, Huynh H, Ahmed N, et al. Toward enteral nutrition for the treatment of pediatric Crohn disease in Canada: A workshop to identify barriers and enablers. Canadian Journal of Gastroenterology and Hepatology. 2015;**29**:351-356

[48] Stewart M, Day AS, Otley A. Physician attitudes and practices of enteral nutrition as primary treatment of paediatric Crohn disease in North America. Journal of Pediatric Gastroenterology and Nutrition. 2011;**52**:38-42. DOI: 10.1097/MPG.0b013e3181e2c724

[49] Whitten KE, Rogers P, Ooi CKY, Day AS. International survey of enteral nutrition protocols used in children with Crohn's disease. Journal of Digestive Diseases. 2012;**13**:107-112. DOI: 10.1111/j.1751-2980.2011.00558.x

[50] Vasseur F, Gower-Rousseau C, Vernier-Massouille G, Dupas JL, Merle V, Merlin B, et al. Nutritional status and growth in pediatric Crohn's disease: A population-based study. The American Journal of Gastroenterology. 2010;**105**:1893-1900. DOI: 10.1038/ajg.2010.20

[51] Ley D, Duhamel A, Behal H, Vasseur F, Sarter H, Michaud L, et al. Growth pattern in paediatric Crohn disease is related to inflammatory status. Journal of Pediatric Gastroenterology and Nutrition. 2016;**63**:637-643. DOI: 10.1097/MPG.0000000000001177

[52] DeBoer MD, Scharf RJ, Leite AM, Férrer A, Havt A, Pinkerton R, et al. Systemic inflammation, growth factors, and linear growth in the setting of infection and malnutrition. Nutrition. 2017;**33**:248-253. DOI: 10.1016/j.nut.2016.06.013

[53] Shamir R, Phillip M, Levine A. Growth retardation in pediatric Crohn's disease. Inflammatory Bowel Diseases. 2007;**13**:620-628. DOI: 10.1002/ibd.20115

[54] Sanderson IR. Growth problems in children with IBD. Nature Reviews. Gastroenterology & Hepatology. 2014;**11**(10):601. DOI: 10.1038/nrgastro.2014.102

[55] Li G, Ren J, Wang G, Hu D, Gu G, Liu S, et al. Preoperative exclusive enteral nutrition reduces the postoperative septic complications of fistulizing Crohn's disease. European Journal of Clinical Nutrition. 2014;**68**:441-446. DOI: 10.1038/ejcn.2014.16

[56] Li Y, Zuo L, Zhu W, Gong J, Zhang W, Gu L, et al. Role of exclusive enteral nutrition in the preoperative optimization of patients with Crohn's disease following immunosuppressive therapy. Medicine (Baltimore). 2015;**94**:e478. DOI: 10.1097/MD.0000000000000478

[57] El-Matary W. Enteral nutrition as a primary therapy of Crohn's disease: The Pediatric perspective. Nutrition in Clinical Practice. 2009;**24**:91-97. DOI: 10.1177/0884533608329660

[58] Alhagamhmad MH, Day AS, Lemberg DA, Leach ST. Exploring and enhancing the anti-inflammatory properties of polymeric formula. Journal of Parenteral and Enteral Nutrition. 2017;**41**:436-445. DOI: 10.1177/0148607115625627

[59] Breese EJ, Michie CA, Nicholls SW, Williams CB, Domizio P, Walker-Smith JA, et al. The effect of treatment on lymphokine-secreting cells in the intestinal mucosa of children with Crohn's disease. Alimentary Pharmacology & Therapeutics 1995;**9**:547-552

[60] Fell JM, Paintin M, Arnaud-Battandier F, Beattie RM, Hollis A, Kitching P, et al. Mucosal healing and a fall in mucosal pro-inflammatory cytokine mRNA induced by a specific oral polymeric diet in paediatric Crohn's disease. Alimentary Pharmacology & Therapeutics. 2000;**14**:281-289

[61] Nahidi L, Corley SM, Wilkins MR, Wei J, Alhagamhmad M, Day AS, et al. The major pathway by which polymeric formula reduces inflammation in intestinal epithelial cells: A microarray-based analysis. Genes & Nutrition. 2015;**10**:29. DOI: 10.1007/s12263-015-0479-x

[62] Guo Z, Gong J, Li Y, Gu L, Cao L, Wang Z, et al. Mucosal MicroRNAs expression profiles before and after exclusive enteral nutrition therapy in adult patients with Crohn's disease. Nutrients. 2016;**8**:519. DOI: 10.3390/nu8080519

[63] de Jong NSH, Leach ST, Day AS. Polymeric formula has direct anti-inflammatory effects on enterocytes in an in VitroModel of intestinal inflammation. Digestive Diseases and Sciences 2007;**52**:2029-2036. DOI: 10.1007/s10620-006-9449-x

[64] Budd GR, Aitchison A, Day AS, Keenan JI. The effect of polymeric formula on enterocyte differentiation. Innate Immunity. 2017;**23**:240-248. DOI: 10.1177/1753425916689333

[65] Giaffer MH, North G, Holdsworth CD. Controlled trial of polymeric versus elemental diet in treatment of active Crohn's disease. Lancet (London, England). 1990;**335**:816-819

[66] Verma S, Brown S, Kirkwood B, Giaffer MH. Polymeric versus elemental diet as primary treatment in active Crohn's disease: A randomized, double-blind trial. The American Journal of Gastroenterology. 2000;**95**:735-739. DOI: 10.1111/j.1572-0241.2000.01527.x

[67] Turner D, Zlotkin S, Shah P, Griffiths A. Omega 3 fatty acids (fish oil) for maintenance of remission in Crohn's disease. In: Turner D, editor. Cochrane Database of Systematic Reviews. Chichester, UK: John Wiley & Sons, Ltd; 2007. p. CD006320. DOI: 10.1002/14651858.CD006320.pub2.

[68] Grogan JL, Casson DH, Terry A, Burdge GC, El-Matary W, Dalzell MA. Enteral feeding therapy for newly diagnosed Pediatric Crohn's disease: A double-blind randomized controlled trial with two years follow-up§. Inflammatory Bowel Diseases. 2012;**18**:246-253. DOI: 10.1002/ibd.21690

[69] Alhagamhmad MH, Day AS, Lemberg DA, Leach ST. An update of the role of nutritional therapy in the management of Crohn's disease. Journal of Gastroenterology. 2012;**47**:872-882. DOI: 10.1007/s00535-012-0617-9

[70] Coëffier M, Marion-Letellier R, Déchelotte P. Potential for amino acids supplementation during inflammatory bowel diseases. Inflammatory Bowel Diseases 2010;**16**:518-524. DOI: 10.1002/ibd.21017

[71] Lecleire S, Hassan A, Marion-Letellier R, Antonietti M, Savoye G, Bole-Feysot C, et al. Combined glutamine and arginine decrease proinflammatory cytokine production by biopsies from Crohn's patients in association with changes in nuclear factor-B and p38 mitogen-activated protein kinase pathways. The Journal of Nutrition. 2008;**138**:2481-2486. DOI: 10.3945/jn.108.099127

[72] Akobeng AK, Miller V, Stanton J, Elbadri AM, Thomas AG. Double-blind randomized controlled trial of glutamine-enriched polymeric diet in the treatment of active Crohn's disease. Journal of Pediatric Gastroenterology and Nutrition. 2000;**30**:78-84

[73] Akobeng AK, Elawad M, Gordon M. Glutamine for induction of remission in Crohn's disease. In: Akobeng AK, editor. Cochrane Database of Systematic Reviews. Vol. 2. Chichester, UK: John Wiley & Sons, Ltd; 2016. p. CD007348. DOI: 10.1002/14651858.CD007348.pub2

[74] Lewis JD, Chen EZ, Baldassano RN, Otley AR, Griffiths AM, Lee D, et al. Inflammation, antibiotics, and diet as environmental stressors of the gut microbiome in pediatric Crohn's disease. Cell Host & Microbe. 2015;**18**:489-500. DOI: 10.1016/j.chom.2015.09.008

[75] Lionetti P, Callegari ML, Ferrari S, Cavicchi MC, Pozzi E, de Martino M, et al. Enteral nutrition and microflora in pediatric Crohn's disease. Journal of Parenteral and Enteral Nutrition. 2005;**29**:S173-S178. DOI: 10.1177/01486071050290S4S173

[76] Leach ST, Mitchell HM, Eng WR, Zhang L, Day AS. Sustained modulation of intestinal bacteria by exclusive enteral nutrition used to treat children with Crohn's disease. Alimentary Pharmacology & Therapeutics. 2008;**28**:724-733

[77] Day AS, Lopez RN. Exclusive enteral nutrition in children with Crohn's disease. World Journal of Gastroenterology. 2015;**21**:6809-6816. DOI: 10.3748/wjg.v21.i22.6809

[78] Gerasimidis K, Bertz M, Hanske L, Junick J, Biskou O, Aguilera M, et al. Decline in presumptively protective gut bacterial species and metabolites are paradoxically associated with disease improvement in pediatric Crohn's disease during enteral nutrition. Inflammatory Bowel Diseases. 2014;**20**:861-871. DOI: 10.1097/MIB.0000000000000023

[79] Quince C, Ijaz UZ, Loman N, Eren AM, Saulnier D, Russell J, et al. Extensive modulation of the fecal metagenome in children with Crohn's disease during exclusive enteral nutrition. The American Journal of Gastroenterology. 2015;**110**:1718-1729. DOI: 10.1038/ajg.2015.357

[80] Kaakoush NO, Day AS, Leach ST, Lemberg DA, Nielsen S, Mitchell HM. Effect of exclusive enteral nutrition on the microbiota of children with newly diagnosed Crohn's disease. Clinical and Translational Gastroenterology. 2015;**6**:e71. DOI: 10.1038/ctg.2014.21

[81] Lee D, Baldassano RN, Otley AR, Albenberg L, Griffiths AM, Compher C, et al. Comparative effectiveness of nutritional and biological therapy in north American children with active Crohn's disease. Inflammatory Bowel Diseases. 2015;**21**:1786-1793. DOI: 10.1097/MIB.0000000000000426

[82] Sarbagili-Shabat C, Sigall-Boneh R, Levine A. Nutritional therapy in inflammatory bowel disease. Current Opinion in Gastroenterology. 2015;**31**:303-308. DOI: 10.1097/MOG.0000000000000178

[83] Harries AD, Jones LA, Danis V, Fifield R, Heatley RV, Newcombe RG, et al. Controlled trial of supplemented oral nutrition in Crohn's disease. Lancet (London, England). 1983;**1**:887-890

[84] Belli DC, Seidman E, Bouthillier L, Weber AM, Roy CC, Pletincx M, et al. Chronic intermittent elemental diet improves growth failure in children with Crohn's disease. Gastroenterology. 1988;**94**:603-610

[85] Wilschanski M, Sherman P, Pencharz P, Davis L, Corey M, Griffiths A. Supplementary enteral nutrition maintains remission in paediatric Crohn's disease. Gut. 1996;**38**:543-548

[86] Kotlyar DS, Lewis JD, Beaugerie L, Tierney A, Brensinger CM, Gisbert JP, et al. Risk of lymphoma in patients with inflammatory bowel disease treated with azathioprine and 6-Mercaptopurine: A meta-analysis. Clinical Gastroenterology and Hepatology. 2015;**13**:847-858.e4. DOI: 10.1016/j.cgh.2014.05.015

[87] Dulai PS, Thompson KD, Blunt HB, Dubinsky MC, Siegel CA. Risks of serious infection or lymphoma with anti-tumor necrosis factor therapy for pediatric inflammatory bowel disease: A systematic review. Clinical Gastroenterology and Hepatology. 2014;**12**:1443-1451. DOI: 10.1016/j.cgh.2014.01.021

[88] Jones VA. Comparison of total parenteral nutrition and elemental diet in induction of remission of Crohn's disease. Long-term maintenance of remission by personalized food exclusion diets. Digestive Diseases and Sciences. 1987;**32**:100S-107S

[89] Verma S, Kirkwood B, Brown S, Giaffer MH. Oral nutritional supplementation is effective in the maintenance of remission in Crohn's disease. Digestive and Liver Disease. 2000;**32**:769-774

[90] Akobeng AK, Thomas AG. Enteral nutrition for maintenance of remission in Crohn's disease. In: Akobeng AK, editor. Cochrane Database of Systematic Reviews. Chichester, UK: John Wiley & Sons, Ltd; 2007. p. CD005984. DOI: 10.1002/14651858.CD005984.pub2

[91] Takagi S, Utsunomiya K, Kuriyama S, Yokoyama H, Takahashi S, Iwabuchi M, et al. Effectiveness of an "half elemental diet" as maintenance therapy for Crohn's disease: A randomized-controlled trial. Alimentary Pharmacology & Therapeutics. 2006;**24**:1333-1340. DOI: 10.1111/j.1365-2036.2006.03120.x

[92] Verma S, Holdsworth CD, Giaffer MH. Does adjuvant nutritional support diminish steroid dependency in Crohn disease? Scandinavian Journal of Gastroenterology. 2001;**36**:383-388

[93] Nakahigashi M, Yamamoto T, Sacco R, Hanai H, Kobayashi F. Enteral nutrition for maintaining remission in patients with quiescent Crohn's disease: Current status and future perspectives. International Journal of Colorectal Disease 2016;**31**:1-7. DOI: 10.1007/s00384-015-2348-x

[94] El-Matary W, Otley A, Critch J, Abou-Setta AM. Enteral feeding therapy for maintaining remission in Crohn's disease: A systematic review. Journal of Parenteral and Enteral Nutrition. 2017;**41**:550-561. DOI: 10.1177/0148607115621051

[95] Johnson T, Macdonald S, Hill SM, Thomas A, Murphy MS. Treatment of active Crohn's disease in children using partial enteral nutrition with liquid formula: A randomised controlled trial. Gut. 2006;**55**:356-361. DOI: 10.1136/gut.2004.062554

[96] Sigall-Boneh R, Pfeffer-Gik T, Segal I, Zangen T, Boaz M, Levine A. Partial enteral nutrition with a Crohn's disease exclusion diet is effective for induction of remission in children and young adults with Crohn's disease. Inflammatory Bowel Diseases. 2014;**20**:1353-1360. DOI: 10.1097/MIB.0000000000000110

[97] Pfeffer-Gik T, Levine A. Dietary clues to the pathogenesis of Crohn's disease. Digestive Diseases. 2014;**32**:389-394. DOI: 10.1159/000358143

Section 5

Pregnancy and Inflammatory Bowel Disease

Chapter 6

Pregnancy and Delivery of Women with IBD

Kateřina Hokerová

Additional information is available at the end of the chapter

http://dx.doi.org/10.5772/intechopen.72827

Abstract

We provide a basic overview of inheritance, fertility and influence of IBD and pregnancy, therapy in pregnancy and childbirth options. A crucial factor for good results is the degree of inflammation at the time of conception and during pregnancy. If the disease is inactive, there is no decrease in fertility and no greater risk of deterioration of disease in pregnancy and pregnancy does not differ from the normal population. The opposite situation occurs if there is a pregnancy at the time of disease activity. Then, in up to 75% of pregnancy courses with big problems, fertility declines, inflammation also worsens and the risk of exacerbations increases during pregnancy. This aggravates the course of pregnancy and childbirth and has a negative effect on the fetus. Therefore, it is necessary to plan for a longer period of disease stabilization and continue chronic medication and not discontinue drugs for the fear of negative impact of medications on fetal development. Commonly used drugs such as aminosalicylates, corticosteroids, immunosuppressants and biological therapy appear to be safe and well tolerated during pregnancy. The method of delivery is different for each individual and depends on the form and location of the inflammation and the preceding operations.

Keywords: inflammatory bowel disease, Crohn's disease, ulcerative colitis, pregnancy, childbirth, breastfeeding

1. Introduction

Inflammatory bowel disease (IBD) is a chronic bowel inflammation of unknown origin, which includes Crohn's disease (CD) and ulcerative colitis (UC). The incidence in our population has increased, the incidence of UC is 10.4/100,000 and the incidence of CD is 5.6/100,000. IBD affects young adults in their fertile age, 50% of patients are diagnosed under the age of 35 and a quarter of patients get pregnant after they have been diagnosed with IBD. Young women are often concerned about the effect of IBD on their fertility, development of the fetus and as well about the effect of the pregnancy on their disease. They are interested in the effect of the chronic medication used during the pregnancy, management of the birth and possibility of breastfeeding. In the past, patients have been advised not to get pregnant, existing strategies of treating IBD makes the pregnancy possible and safe for the mother and the child.

2. Genetics and IBD

IBD is multifactorially determined. The risk for a child with a parent with an IBD is 2–13 times higher than the risk in the normal population [1]. A child of a parent with IBD has a 5% risk for CD and a 1.6% for UC. If both parents have IBD, the risk increases up to 37% [2, 3].

3. Fertility and IBD

Infertility of women with IBD ranges between 7 and 12%, which is in line with the normal population [4–7]. The fertility can decrease with the following conditions:

- An active inflammation (can affect the Fallopian tubes and the ovaries, in the perianal area it can cause dyspareunia)
- Surgery before the pregnancy (IPAA—ileo pouch anal anastomosis—is connected with lower fertility because of scarring in the area around the adnexae)
- Medication that affects men's fertility such as methotrexate, sulfasalazine [1, 9, 10]

4. The effects of IBD on pregnancy

Multiple studies on the effects of IBD on pregnancy, development and growth of the fetus, have come to a conflicting conclusions most likely due to disparate conditions of the individual studies. All the studies agree that the key factor for a successful pregnancy is a function of whether the disease is active at the time of conception. Patients with an inactive IBD (minimum 12 months without clinical, laboratory and endoscopic signs of an active inflammatory process) are not in a higher risk of bad perinatological results. On the other hand, if the disease is active, up to 75% of pregnancies are connected with a high number of problems and relatively high risk of abortion, preterm birth or hypotrophy of the fetus. Therefore, it is necessary to plan the pregnancy while the disease is in remission [1, 4–6, 8]. The activity of the disease at the time of conception leads to a higher risk of fetal loss and preterm deliveries. Also, activity of the disease during the pregnancy is associated with lower fetal weight and as well with a preterm delivery [1, 3, 8, 9, 10]. Pregnancy loss affects 12.2% of patients with IBD as compared to 9.9% in the normal population. Miscarriages are more common in cases where

http://dx.doi.org/10.5772/intechopen.72827

the patient has an intestinal resection before the pregnancy. The length of the resected tissue and activity of the disease are proportional to a higher risk of miscarriage [6]. The percentage of preterm deliveries (<g.h. 37) is around 8% in the Czech Republic in the normal population, studies describe higher risk of preterm deliveries in the group of people with IBD, the risk is 1.87 times higher, which is 11.5–16% [6]. The risk of low fetal weight (<2500 g) is two times higher, which is explained by undernourishment of the mother in the time of relapse, especially if there are repeated exacerbations in the course of the pregnancy. This occurs more often in diseased with the CD than the UC, Although some studies have found a connection between congenital malformations (especially a cleft palate and malformations of the urinary tract) and the mother's UC, this suspicion was not confirmed in extensive studies. Most of the studies show that IBD is not connected with a risk of congenital malformations. The rate of malformations ranges between 1 and 4.8% of newborns, which is the same range as in the normal population. More serious malformations were more often found in a group with a severe course of the disease during the pregnancy compared to the ones in relapse. After considering the grade of disease, no study was able to prove that any medication used (corticoids, azathioprine and mesalazine) affects the result of pregnancy [5].

5. The effect of pregnancy on IBD

There is no proof to suggest that pregnancy worsens the disease; therefore, there is no reason to end the pregnancy. On the contrary, there are studies that have demonstrated positive effects and long-term improvement of IBD (impact of the pregnancy on the immune system) shown decrease of relapses in the following 3 years [2]. Development of IBD during the pregnancy is correlated with the activity of disease at the time of conception. If the disease is inactive at the time of conception, then the pregnancy goes without bigger problems in the majority of the diseased, only around one-third of patients have a relapse during the pregnancy, which is the same number as in a group of nonpregnant women in the course of 9 months. In two-thirds of the patients, the disease stays in inactive state during the whole pregnancy [1, 4, 6, 8]. On the other hand, if the IBD is active at the time of conception, two-thirds of the patients have a persistent disease and even an aggravation of the disease. Therapy plays an important role in pregnancy by keeping the disease in remission; therefore, it is recommended that the therapy should not be stopped due to the fear of side effects to pregnancy.

6. Therapy in pregnancy

The majority of the drugs used for the treatment of IBD are considered to be safe during the pregnancy and breastfeeding [3]. Analysis of 19 retrospective studies has shown that the medication commonly used for therapy of IBD (aminosalicylates—ASA, corticoids, immunosuppressants and immunotherapy) does not significantly increase the incidence of stillborn, ectopic pregnancy, hypotrophy of the fetus or miscarriage. While using these drugs, the congenital anomalies were more often seen, which is probably connected to the activity of the disease and not to the therapy. Both methotrexate and thalidomide are clearly contraindicated [1].

If the therapy is able to keep the disease inactive, it is recommended not to stop and continue the therapy during the whole pregnancy because the benefits outweigh the risks of the conservative therapy and the danger of relapse after completing the therapy.

7. The mode of delivery

The percentage (44%) of the Cesarean section is higher in the group of patients with IBD than in normal population [3]. Recent population studies from Sweden have shown that women with the UC without any surgery in the past had two times higher risk of elective Cesarean section, even though vaginal birth is the safest way for the mother and the child. Additional studies have also shown that the Cesarean sections are mostly performed on the basis of patient's or the doctor's preference, but not from a real indication. Even though some doctors think that all the patients with IBD should have a Cesarean section, it seems reasonable to make the vaginal birth possible for the women with inactive or in the moderate stage of the disease. The decision about the mode of the delivery should be strictly individual and it should be an agreement among the mother, the obstetrician, the gastroenterologist and the surgeon [6].

Cesarean section is definitely indicated when there is an active perianal disease with abscesses and fistulas or active rectal disease (proctitis in UC and CD) with consideration of the protection of the anal sphincter. IPAA or ileorectal anastomosis is considered as a relative indication for the Cesarean section, the guidelines about the mode of delivery after IPAA are not uniform, and both ways are described. With a consideration of a protection of the anal sphincter and keeping the pouch continence, the Cesarean section is preferred. Patients with the IPAA have, due to the surgery, a border continence of stool and that is closely related to an intact sphincter and the function of the pelvic floor. The function of the pouch is affected already in the third trimester and it goes back to the original shape during 6 months after the delivery. In the vaginal birth, the pudendal nerves can be affected due to the pressure in the second stage of labor or in the forceps delivery, which can lead to more frequent stools. In the long-term observation (5 years), it is observed that after the vaginal birth, the function of the pouch worsens faster especially in the births with the higher risks of obstetric injuries (instrumental labor, episiotomy, the fetal weight above 4000 g, emergent Cesarean section, second stage of labor longer than 2 h) In the majority of the patients, the primary Cesarean section is chosen. Other reason for that is as well the emergency Cesarean section from the obstetrics indication can be very risky because of abdominal adhesions after previous surgeries [1, 3, 9, 10]. Vaginal birth should be allowed only to women without the signs of rectal and perianal forms of the disease [6]. Traumatic changes of the perianal area can be a cause of long-term festering complications or fistulas, preforming of episiotomy can induce the perianal lesions in the future course of the disease in 20% [5]. If the woman with IBD has a vaginal birth, it is appropriate to avoid episiotomy; however, it is better to perform an episiotomy than a spontaneous uncontrollable damage. Vaginal birth is also possible in the patients with colostomy or ileostomy and it is not associated with a higher risk of the complications with the stomies [1, 6].

8. Conclusion

IBD affects women in the fertile age with consequences to their fertility, pregnancy and breastfeeding. The disease and the pregnancy affect each other, and the development of the disease and the pregnancy is determined by the activity of inflammation at the time of conception. Patients who are in remission at the time of conception will most likely stay in the remission during the pregnancy. On the other hand, 70% of the patients with an active inflammation at the time of conception will stay in that shape or even get worse during the pregnancy. Women with an active IBD are at a higher risk of adverse results of the pregnancy, whereas the women with inactive disease can expect normal course and good results of the pregnancy. That is why it is crucial to plan their pregnancy during remission, and not to cut out the anti-inflammatory and immunosuppressant therapy put in place before the pregnancy. Most of the medication used in treatment of IBD is considered to be safe at the time of pregnancy and breastfeeding, but more studies are needed. Patients with IBD can have vaginal delivery, whereas patients with the perianal lesions, patients with affected rectum and patients after the reconstructive surgery with IPAA should deliver by the Cesarean section.

Author details

Kateřina Hokerová

Address all correspondence to: zavorova@nemocnice-horovice.cz

Nemocnice Hořovice, Hořovice, Czech Republic

References

[1] Van der Woude CJ. ECCO Guidelines/Consensus Paper. The second European evidenced-based consensus on reproduction and pregnancy in inflammatory bowel disease. Journal of Crohn's and Colitis. 2015;**9**(2):107-124. Available from: https://www.ecco-ibd.eu/images/6_Publication/6_3_ECCO%20Guidelines/FINAL_MASTER_JCC_Online_PulishedVersion_PregnancyGuidelines_2015_Doi101093_jju006.pdf

[2] Kment M. Idiopatické střevní záněty v graviditě. Interní medicína pro praxi. 2008;**10**(7a8):333-335

[3] Kwan LY, Mahadevan U. Inflammatory bowel disease and pregnancy: An update. Expert Review of Clinical Immunology. 2010;**6**(4):643-657

[4] Alstead EM, Nelson-Piercy C. Inflammatory bowel disease in pregnancy. 2013. Available from: http://www.ncbi.nlm.nih.gov/pmc/articles/PMC1774968/

[5] Kment M. Choroby gastrointestinálního traktu v graviditě. Triton. 2003:43-61

[6] Lukáš K, Pařízek A. Idiopatické střevní záněty a těhotenství. Časopis lékařů českých. 2010;**149**:163-172

[7] Pintérová Kolesárová M, Pintér M. Vliv idiopatického střevního zánětu na interval potřebný pro početí pacientek. Česká Gynekologie 2008;**732**:109-112

[8] Ferguson ChB. Inflammatory bowel disease in pregnancy. British Medical Journal. 2008;**337**(a427). Available from: http://dx.doi.org/10.1136/bmj.39566.681458.BE (Published July 2008); http://www.bmj.com/content/337/bmj.39566.681458.BE

[9] Peppercon MA, Mahadevan U. Fertility, pregnancy and nursing in inflammatory bowel disease. 2017. Available from: http://www.uptodate.com/contents/fertility-pregnancy and-nursing-in-inflammatory-bowel-disease

[10] Peppercon MA, Mahadevan U. Patient information: Inflammatory bowel disease and pregnancy. 2017. Available from: http://www.uptodate.com/contents/inflammatory-boweldisease-and-pregnancy-beyond-the-basics